A Colour Atlas of

Allergic Skin Disorders

Rino Cerio, BSc, MB, BS, MRCP
Consultant Dermatologist
The Royal London Hospital
London, England

William F. Jackson, MA, MB, BChir, MRCP
Formerly Honorary Consultant in Allergy
Department of Medicine
Guy's Hospital
London, England

Wolfe Publishing Limited

Acknowledgements
We gratefully acknowledge the help of a number of colleagues who allowed us to borrow illustrations to fill the gaps in our own collections:

A. Bloom, J. Ireland, P. Watkins (**15**); A.C. Boyle (**138, 186**); T.R. Bull (**71, 72**); G.S.J. Chessell, M.J. Jamieson, R. A. Morton, J.C. Petrie, H.M.A. Towler (**113, 114, 127**); G.M. Cochrane, P.J. Rees (**41, 47**); W.B. Conolly (**139, 140, 141**); D.C. Evered, R. Hall (**110, 111, 227**); R. Fulton (**76**); T.P. Habif (**14, 25, 31, 32, 56, 118, 122, 123, 124, 130, 178**); P. Hall-Smith (**160**); F.G.J. Hayhoe, R.J. Flemans (**45, 46**); D.G. James, P.R. Studdy (**143, 144**); A. Kamal, J.C. Brocklehurst (**115, 136**); G.M. Levene, C.D. Calnan (**3, 4, 16, 57, 59, 88, 133, 180, 181, 191, 203**); G.M. Levene, S.K. Goolamali (**6, 80, 89, 179, 184, 204**); R.D.G. Milner, S.M. Herber (**53**); W. Peters (**77**); R. E. Pounder, M.C. Allison, A.P. Dhillon (**10, 104, 106, 131, 199**); C.V. Ruckley (**142**); L.M. Shapiro, K.M. Fox (**19**); R. Staughton (**11**); L. A. Stone, E. M. Lindfield, S. Robertson (**26, 27, 28, 29, 30, 36, 37, 38, 197, 231, 232, 233, 234, 236, 237**); W.R. Tyldesley (**12, 52**); W.L. Weston, A.T. Lane (**58, 92, 93, 94, 119, 176**); G. Williams (**129**); A. Wisdom (**168**); V. Wright, A.R. Harvey (**43, 44, 137**); and M. Zatouroff (**9, 109**).

Copyright © 1992 Wolfe Publishing Ltd
Published by Wolfe Publishing Ltd, 1992
Printed by BPCC Hazell Books Ltd, Aylesbury, England
ISBN 0 7234 1797 0

All rights reserved. No production, copy or transmission of this publication may be made without written permission.

No part of this publication may be reproduced, copied or transmitted save with written permission or in accordance with the provisions of the Copyright Act 1956 (as amended), or under the terms of any licence permitting limited copying issued by the Copyright Licensing Agency, 33–34 Alfred Place, London, WC1E 7DP.

Any person who does any unauthorised act in relation to this publication may be liable to criminal prosecution and civil claims for damages.

A CIP catalogue record for this book is available from the British Library.

For full details of Wolfe titles please write to Wolfe Publishing Ltd, 2–16 Torrington Place, London WC1E 7LT, England.

Contents

Preface	4
1. Diagnosis in Allergic Skin Disease	5
History	5
Physical examination	8
Is this an allergic skin disorder?	14
Allergic skin disease and atopy	15
Hyper-reactivity	16
A cautionary note	16
2. Mechanisms of Allergic Skin Reactions	17
The innate immune system	17
The adaptive immune system	17
The skin immune system	19
Abnormalities of the immune system	20
3. Investigation of Skin Allergy	23
Patch tests	23
Skin prick tests	27
Skin biopsy	28
Investigations on peripheral blood	29
Other investigations	32
4. Skin Disorders Associated with Immediate Allergic Reactions	33
Urticaria	33
Reactive erythemas	41
Atopic eczema	42
Allergic rhinitis	44
Nasal polyps	46
Immediate allergic reactions in the eye	46
Insect sting allergy	48
5. Skin Disorders Associated with Autoantibodies	49
Immunobullous disorders	49
Non-bullous dermatoses	54
Organ-specific autoimmune disorders with skin manifestations	62
6. Skin Disorders Associated with Immune Complexes	65
Vasculitis	65
Vasculitis with granuloma formation	76
7. Skin Disorders Associated with Delayed Allergic Reactions	81
Contact allergic dermatitis	81
Contact irritant dermatitis	91
Photoallergy	92
Atopic eczema and immune mechanisms	92
Auto-eczema and immune mechanisms	92
Auto-eczematisation	92
Granulomas	93
8. Photosensitivity and Photoallergy	97
Drugs and photosensitivity	101
Differential diagnosis	102
Management	102
9. Allergy to Drugs and Food	103
Drug reactions in the skin	103
Food allergy and the skin	109
10. Eczema and Dermatitis	113
Exogenous dermatitis	114
Endogenous dermatitis	114
Unclassified dermatitis	120
11. Management of Allergic Skin Disorders	123
Type I reactions	123
Type II reactions	123
Type III reactions	123
Type IV reactions	123
Index	127

Preface

Skin disorders are a common presenting complaint in general practice and are a frequent occurrence in patients presenting to most medical (and surgical) specialists. Many of these disorders develop wholly or partly through immunological or allergic mechanisms, and – although these mechanisms are not always fully understood – it is clear that 'allergy', in the broad sense of the term, plays an important role in many dermatoses. Patients are, perhaps, more frequently correct in attributing skin problems to 'allergy' than we realise; and many doctors are still rather puzzled by this wide group of skin diseases.

In this book we use the term 'allergy' synonymously with hypersensitivity reactions, as defined by Gell and Coombs, and we group allergic skin disorders according to Gell and Coombs' classification, to clarify their mechanisms. Not all allergic skin disorders fit neatly into this classification, however – atopic eczema, for example, undoubtedly involves more than one mechanism. We include most skin disorders in which allergy or hypersensitivity reactions play a major role, but we have excluded some common disorders – such as psoriasis – in which such reactions are probably not of primary importance (though they may yet prove to have a significant role). We have also excluded the dermatological manifestations of immunodeficiency states, and most conditions where the primary disorder is known to be infective in origin; though – as we acknowledge – it is still possible that infection may have an important *initiating* role in some of the disorders we have included.

We have used the terms 'eczema' and 'dermatitis' as synonyms throughout the book, but we have usually referred to 'atopic eczema' and 'contact dermatitis'. Our choice of terminology has the advantage of conforming with common everyday usage in many centres; but it does not imply any major difference of opinion with those who prefer to use the term 'dermatitis' for both atopic and contact skin disorders.

We hope that this book will be helpful to all those involved in the care of patients with allergic skin disorders, but our principal target is the generalist rather than the specialist. Specialist dermatologists may find the colour illustrations and the immunological classification interesting and useful, but our text is aimed squarely at the more general medical reader. We have not tried to compete with large textbooks on dermatology – rather, we have aimed to present a simple practical overview, with an emphasis on the visual aspects of diagnosis and management. Many excellent textbooks provide the interested reader with more information on the conditions we have included, and on their management.

Many of the clinical photographs in the book came from our own collections, but others have been generously loaned by friends or colleagues in this country and overseas. They are acknowledged in detail elsewhere, and we thank them all for their help. We affectionately dedicate the book to Soraya, Alexander, Olivia and Rebecca Cerio, and to Barbara, Clare, and Ian Jackson, who all provided constant encouragement during its relatively brief but intensive gestation period.

Rino Cerio
William F Jackson
London, England

1 Diagnosis in Allergic Skin Disease

Allergic reactions may occur throughout the body, but their manifestations are more obvious in the skin than elsewhere. As a major interface of the body with the environment, the skin is also a focus for localised allergic reactions. Foreign antigens are recognised by specialised skin cells (mainly Langerhans cells), and may trigger antibody production and an inflammatory response involving lymphocytes, macrophages, polymorphs, and the release of cytokines and mediators.

The skin consists of a number of layers and tissue components which have a variety of functions. A wide spectrum of allergic skin reactions may occur in the different layers and subcomponents of human skin, and their clinical manifestations reflect – among other things – the layers in which the reactions occur **(1, 2)**.

History

In a skin disease, the patient's history and the findings on examination often provide valuable clues as to the probable underlying diagnosis. The important aspects to be considered in examining the patient's history include:

- A description of the events that accompany the onset of skin lesions.
- The progression of individual lesions, including the role of aggravating and relieving factors.
- Is the condition acute, chronic, or recurrent?
- Is there a relevant previous or family history?
- Is the skin disorder associated with symptoms or signs of other disease?
- Is there an obvious relationship to drug therapy or foods?

Other key points in dermatological history-taking are summarised in *Table 1*.

Table 1. *Outline of dermatological history.*	
History of present skin problem	• Duration • Site of onset, details of spread • Itching? • Burning/soreness? • Wet, dry, scaly, blisters?
Past history of skin disorders	• Urticaria • Eczema • Psoriasis
Past general medical history	• Atopy – asthma, hay fever • Systemic disorder
Social and occupational history	• Work • Hobbies • Foreign travel

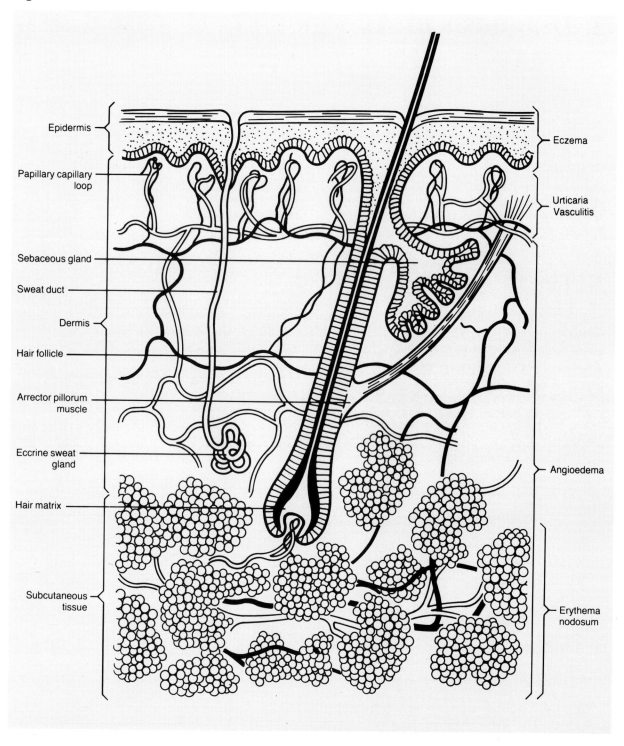

1 The anatomy of the full thickness of the skin in section. Note the layers in which different allergic skin disorders occur.

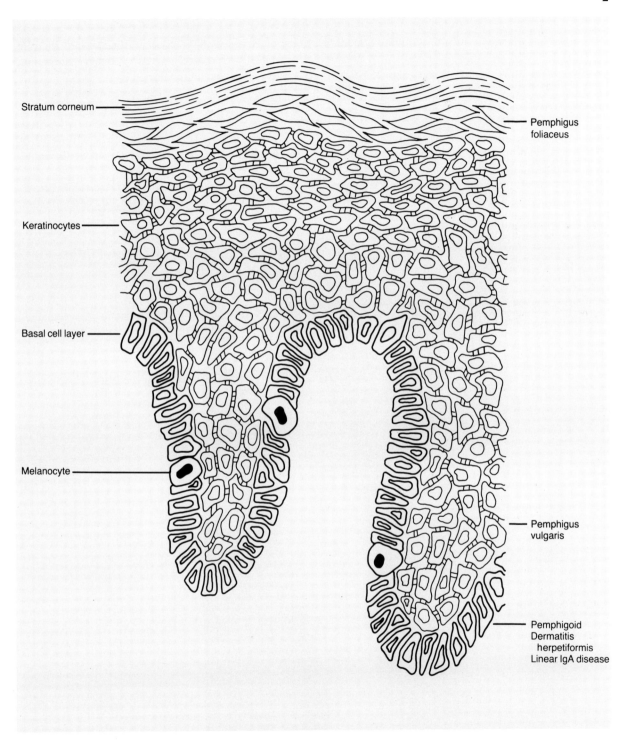

2 The anatomy of the epidermis. Note the layers in which different allergic skin disorders occur.

Physical Examination

The accurate diagnosis of allergic skin disorders requires careful examination of the patient. The skin, hair, nails, and mucous membranes should be fully exposed and well lit. Skin lesions should then be examined with special reference to their distribution, arrangement, and morphology.

Distribution

The distribution of lesions offers important clues for diagnosis. The presence or absence of symmetry helps to distinguish 'internal' or endogenous causes from 'external' or exogenous causes. Exogenous disease, including infection as well as contact allergic skin disorders, often presents in a unilateral or asymmetrical distribution, whereas endogenous disease is commonly symmetrical.

Endogenous allergic eruptions include atopic eczema (**3, 4**), dermatitis herpetiformis (**5**), and vasculitis (**6**).

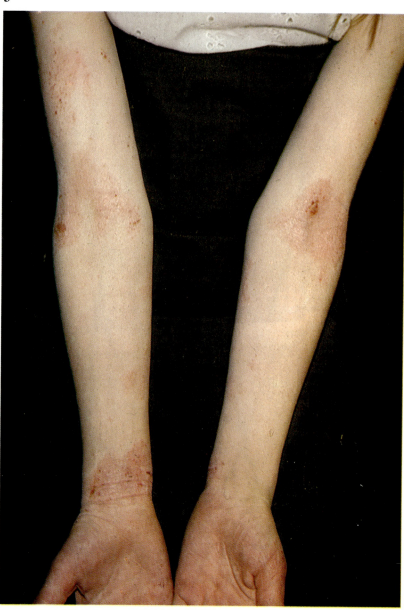

3 Atopic eczema classically occurs in the body flexures and is usually symmetrically distributed. In contrast to other allergic skin disorders, eczema affects the epidermis, and its appearance is modified by scratching and secondary infection.

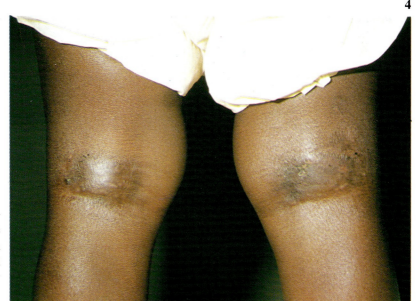

4 Atopic eczema in a dark-skinned child. As in **3**, the eczema occurs in the skin flexures, but in dark-skinned patients chronic lesions typically become hyperpigmented.

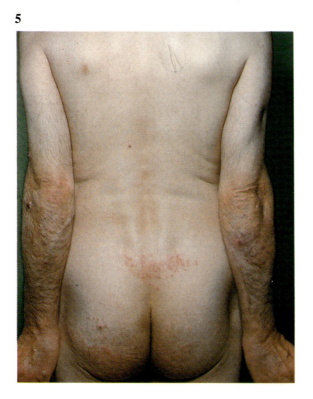

5 Dermatitis herpetiformis is a subepidermal cytotoxic autoimmune disorder with a classical distribution, as shown in this patient. It commonly presents as clusters of vesicles affecting the extensor surfaces of the elbows, lower back, buttocks, and scalp. The distribution is usually symmetrical, and the condition is often misdiagnosed as eczema. Skin biopsy, including immunofluorescence, confirms the diagnosis.

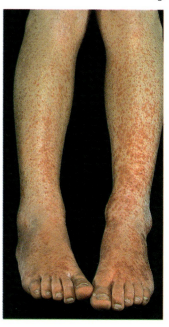

6 Vasculitis that affects the small vessels is often symmetrical and occurs in gravity-dependent areas, such as the legs. Due to inflammation of the vessels in the epidermis, vasculitic purpura is palpable. Rarely, it may blister or even ulcerate. Immunofluorescence studies show immune-complex deposition in the post-capillary venule.

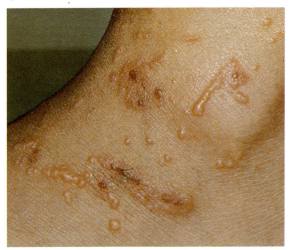

Exogenous allergic eruptions include contact allergic dermatoses; for example, those due to nickel, poison ivy (**7**), perfume, topical medicaments, and other substances (**8**).

7 Contact allergic dermatitis to poison ivy and related plants is a common problem in North America. This 15-year-old boy presented with linear eczematous lesions on his ankle, after walking through a wooded area.

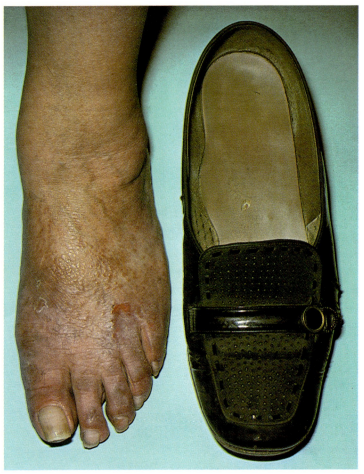

8 Shoe dermatitis is an example of contact allergy (Type IV). The distribution of the dermatitis gives an obvious clue to its cause. Patch testing is required to confirm the allergen. In this case, patch testing showed a positive reaction to potassium dichromate, which is used as a tanning agent in curing leather. Other possible causes of shoe dermatitis include dyes or resins.

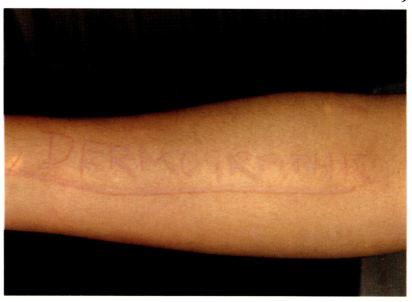

9 Dermographism is a common form of physical urticaria, which results from the extravasation of fluid around the upper dermal vessels in response to mild scratching. Urticaria may occur on any part of the body surface and in the dermographic patient can be easily elicited by the clinician (see **25**).

The distribution of lesions, however, does not always distinguish between endogenous and exogenous causes. For example, dermographism may be provoked asymmetrically, though the underlying hyper-reactivity is symmetrical (**9**); and conditions such as erythema multiforme (**10**) may be symmetrical, though the precipitating factors originate from outside the body.

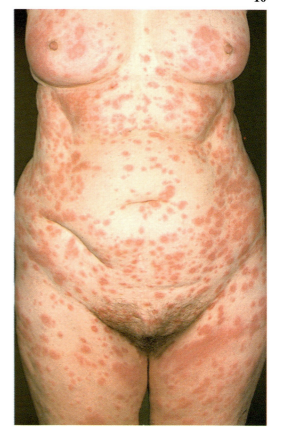

10 Erythema multiforme as a component of the Stevens–Johnson syndrome. This middle-aged lady has a widespread symmetrical eruption composed of erythematous target-like lesions. She also had mucosal involvement, with ulceration in her mouth and vagina. She later developed subepidermal blistering in some of the lesions. The patient had been prescribed sulphasalazine for ulcerative colitis. Sulphasalazine is sulphapyridine covalently bound to 5-aminosalicylic acid, and the rash is usually attributable to the sulphonamide component of the drug. New drugs, such as mesalazine and olsalazine, contain only the aspirin-like moiety, and are very unlikely to cause this allergic reaction.

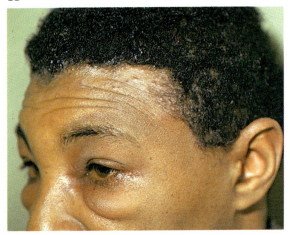

11 An acute eczematous facial eruption with oedema, as seen around the eyes in this patient, can be the result of allergic contact dermatitis (Type IV reaction) to contact allergens, such as hair dye. The clue in this case is weeping dermatitis of the scalp. Patch testing showed a positive reaction to the black hair dye paraphenylenediamine.

Sometimes the location of lesions can offer clues to aetiology; for example, in some forms of contact allergic dermatitis (**11**) or in photosensitivity reactions. Negative as well as positive findings should be noted; for example, in photosensitivity, areas not exposed to light are spared.

Even where the morphology is similar, distribution can be helpful in the differential diagnosis of allergic and non-allergic skin disease. For example, seborrhoeic dermatitis typically affects the scalp, forehead, eyebrows, nasolabial folds, and central chest; whereas atopic eczema affects the flexures, especially the antecubital and popliteal fossae. Pityriasis rosea affects predominantly the trunk, with the long axis of the oval lesions along the lines of cleavage; scabies affects the wrists, finger webs, genitalia (in men), and breasts (in women); erythema nodosum affects the extensor surfaces of the legs and only rarely the arms. It is always important to inspect the mouth (**12**) and the nails (**13**).

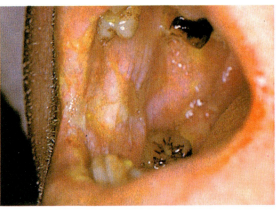

12 Pemphigus vulgaris affecting the oral mucosa. In this condition, cytotoxic autoantibodies produce an intra-epidermal split with blistering. The process affects both the skin – most commonly in a symmetrical distribution on the trunk – and the mucous membranes, including the mouth.

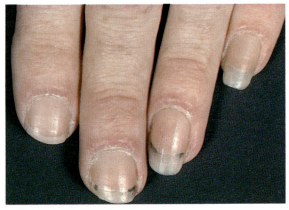

13 Nail fold erythema and telangiectasia with ragged cuticles. This clinical appearance can accompany non-organ-specific autoimmune disorders, such as systemic lupus erythematosus or, as in this patient, dermatomyositis. The appearance is symmetrical, and usually affects most nails. The mechanism is unclear, but cytotoxic autoantibodies can be found in these patients.

Arrangement of lesions

It is important to note the pattern or relationship of nearby, but not confluent, lesions. Typical patterns include clusters [the grouped vesicles of dermatitis herpetiformis (**14**)], beading [closely set, but not confluent, papules in a linear or circular arrangement, as in granuloma annulare (**15**)], reticular (lattice or net-like arrangement in vesicular lesions), and linearity (as in bed-bug bites).

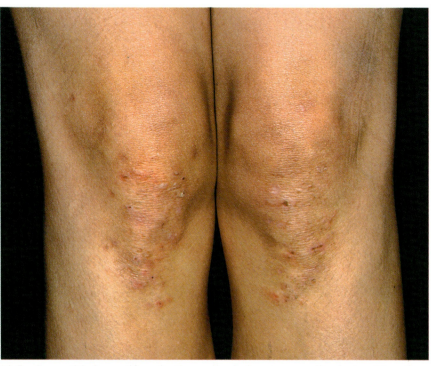

14 In dermatitis herpetiformis, the vesilar lesions are usually clustered together. The symmetrical lesions, seen on the knees of this patient, are typical. Most of the vesicles have been excoriated by scratching.

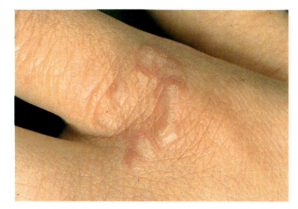

15 Beading of lesions in a circular arrangement is typical of granuloma annulare, as seen in these lesions on the finger of a diabetic patient. Histologically, the lesions show a dermal focus of palasading histiocytes and/or macrophages, often surrounding areas of collagen degeneration. The cause of the disorder is obscure, and allergic processes are not known to be involved.

Table 2. *Terminology used to describe skin lesions.*

Nature of lesion	Size	
	Small (<0.5 cm)	Large (>0.5 cm)
Flat area	Macule	Patch
Elevated and solid	Papule (or papilloma)	Nodule Plaque (flatter but > 2.0 cm)
Fluid-filled	Vesicle	Bulla
Pus-filled	Pustule	Abscess
Vascular	Petechia (pin-head size)	Ecchymosis
	Purpura (up to 2 mm in diameter)	Haematoma
Dermal oedema	Weal (any size)	Angioedema (if subcutaneous tissue involved)

Morphology of lesions

The morphology of individual lesions should be noted, including their size, colour, consistency, configuration, margination, and surface characteristics *(Table 2)*.

Is this an Allergic Skin Disorder?

To the layman, 'allergy' means intolerance or hypersensitivity to an external substance or stimulus, or sometimes even a skin eruption of any cause **(16)**. To the specialist, an allergic reaction is usually defined as a hypersensitivity reaction based on an immunological mechanism, but even so the term 'allergy' can mean different things to different specialists.

In this book the term 'allergy' is regarded as synonymous with immunological hypersensitivity, in accordance with the classification of Gell and Coombs (*Table 3* and see Chapter 2). The 'allergic' skin disorders described herein are those in which there is evidence for a specific immune or allergic response which is associated with or causes the skin disorder.

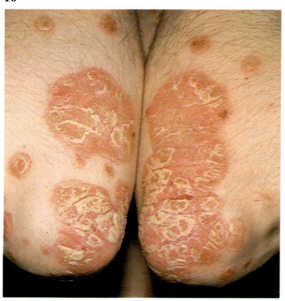

16

Table 3. *Gell and Coombs' classification of hypersensitivity states.*

Type I	Anaphylactic, IgE-mediated, or immediate type
Type II	Cytotoxic Type III Immune complex
Type IV	Cell-mediated or delayed type

16 Psoriasis is a common dermatological condition, and patients may sometimes misinterpret it as an 'allergy' 30% of patients have a family history of the condition, but its overall cause is unknown. The hyperkeratotic psoriatic plaques on the extensor surfaces of the elbows are typical. The lesions are sharply circumscribed, red, and covered in silvery scales. The elbows and knees are commonly involved, and the lesions are usually symmetrical.

Human existence inevitably involves contact not only with different pathogens, but also with a variety of other foreign substances which are potentially antigenic. Killing pathogens requires the immune system to be capable of many different responses and it is, perhaps, not surprising that a proportion of the population develop 'inappropriate' immune responses to harmless foreign proteins or 'allergens'.

It is not always easy to differentiate between allergic and non-allergic skin disorders at the clinical level; and even at the level of basic science the distinction can be blurred. Even where an allergic reaction is the undoubted basis of a dermatological disorder, the manifestations of the disorder may be modified by many internal and external influences, including genetic and psychological factors, infections and other diseases, drug therapy, and a range of local and general environmental influences (**17**).

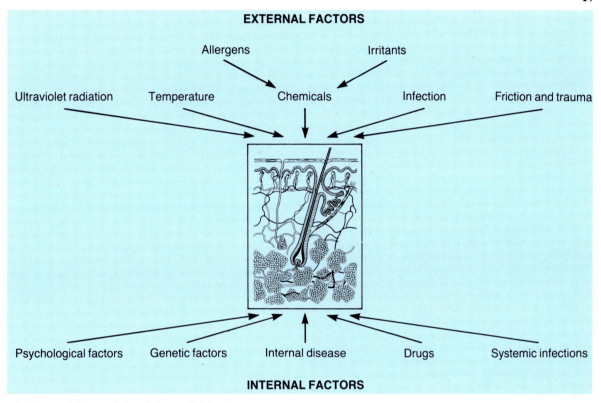

17 The multifactorial aetiology of skin disease.

Allergic Skin Disease and Atopy

There is increasing evidence that some dermatological disorders are caused by a complex interplay of more than one mechanism.

Multiple immunological mechanisms may be involved in some processes, and these may interact with genetic, environmental, and other factors. Two common but quite different 'allergic' skin disorders, urticaria (Chapter 4) and contact allergic eczema/dermatitis (Chapter 7), can, for example, be related to other endogenous or exogenous factors. They may also develop after prolonged exposure of the immune system to the allergens (an induction period).

An acquired specific alteration in the capacity to react to antigens is fundamental to the mechanism of allergy, and the tendency towards pathological immune reactions may be inherited. A genetic predisposition exists for atopy and for some of the autoimmune diseases (Chapters 5 and 6). In 1923, Cooke and Coca proposed the term atopy for those clinical forms of allergy (eczema, asthma, and hay fever) in which the individual has an inherited predisposition to become sensitised. Later, the presence of a high circulating 'reagin' or IgE was added to the definition as another characteristic of atopy.

Hyper-reactivity

It is characteristic of many of the skin diseases described here that a series of stimuli which cause little or no reaction in normal subjects may result in symptoms such as pruritus in patients. This abnormal responsiveness may result from a specific allergy, but recently it has become clear that an increased non-specific responsiveness of the skin – hyper-reactivity – is also of considerable importance. There is a parallel here with the recognition of the importance of non-specific bronchial hyper-reactivity in patients with asthma.

A number of skin diseases are associated with abnormal reactivity, especially to pruritic stimuli. Patients with atopic eczema, for example, have an abnormal response to injection of the para-sympathetic neurotransmitter acetylcholine. In normal subjects this produces vasodilatation and an erythematous flare, but in hyper-reactive eczema patients it produces blanching. This so-called paradoxical vascular response can also be demonstrated by scratching the skin, when the patient develops 'white dermographism' (**18**). A subgroup of patients with chronic urticaria react abnormally to mechanical stress; and some react to various physical stimuli, for example, those with dermographism and those whose urticaria develops in response to cold, pressure, ultraviolet light, and exercise.

The basis of non-specific hyper-reactivity is poorly understood. At best it is described as a result of an autonomic imbalance, which may have both adrenergic and cholinergic components, especially in atopic patients.

18

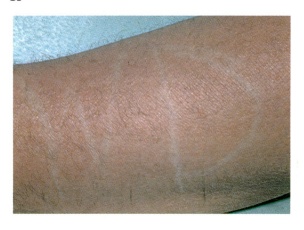

18 White dermographism. This young patient has extensive unstable atopic eczema. In normal individuals, scratching the skin produces an erythematous response: but in eczematous patients a 'paradoxial' response may occur – so-called white dermographism. This response is quite different from patients with physical urticaria (see **9**).

A Cautionary Note

The term *skin allergy* is often poorly understood by the general public, and sometimes even by doctors. Genuine allergy is a specific hypersensitivity involving immunological mechanisms. Allergic rhinitis is a good example of an obvious allergic reaction, where pollen and/or house dust mite excreta are the known allergens. Skin rashes can develop as a consequence of a drug allergy, for example, to penicillin. However, an adverse skin reaction to contact irritants, such as detergents, is often misinterpreted as allergy. *The features of many allergic skin disorders can be mimicked by non-allergic disease.*

Many skin reactions are good examples of immune mechanisms at work, but beware of accepting that immunological events are the prime cause of any disorder until it is completely understood. If *Treponema pallidum* had not been discovered, syphilis might now be classified as an autoimmune disorder!

It is likely that infective or other provoking factors will, in time, be found to account for the immunological reactions which underlie some of the skin disorders described here.

Allergic skin disorders may be secondary to other treatable diseases.

2 Mechanisms of Allergic Skin Reactions

Many allergic skin reactions are good indicators of immune mechanisms at work (**19**). The immune system functions in the skin, just as it does in any other organ of the body.

The body's immune system is divided functionally into innate (non-specific) and adaptive (specific) components.

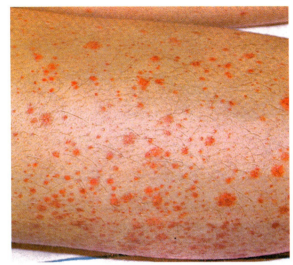

19 Vasculitis may occur in many parts of the body, but its dermatological manifestations often provide the first clue to the underlying systemic immunological processes. This patient has leucocytoclastic vasculitis. The typical purpuric, vasculitic rash was palpable – the result of inflammation of the microcirculation as a consequence of immune complex deposition in the vessel walls (a Type III allergic reaction).

The Innate Immune System

The first line of defence of the body against infection is provided by the innate immune system, which consists of a range of physical, chemical, and cellular mechanisms (*Table 4*). These mechanisms are active in all normal individuals, and prevent most potential infections caused by pathogens. But they are not specific, and they are not enhanced by repeated infection.

Table 4. *The innate immune system.*

Biochemical defences	Physical defences
Lysozyme in mucosal secretions	Skin
Complement	Cilia in respiratory tract
Acute phase proteins – e.g. Interferon and C-reactive protein (CRP)	Mucus
Sebaceous gland secretions	*Cellular defences*
Commensal gut and vaginal organisms	Phagocytes
Spermine in semen	Natural killer (NK) cells
Acid in stomach	

The Adaptive Immune System

The adaptive immune system comes into play when the innate immune system has failed to deal with a foreign antigen. The adaptive system involves both cellular and humoral mechanisms, and is characterised by specific immunological memory, so that a repeat exposure to the organism or antigen at a later date provokes an enhanced immune response. This enhanced response produces a life-long immunity to diseases such as diphtheria and measles following the first infection, and can be said to be 'appropriate' in these circumstances. Clinical allergy is concerned mainly with the effects of the apparently *inappropriate* function of the adaptive immune system (though abnormalities of the innate immune system are sometimes also of significance).

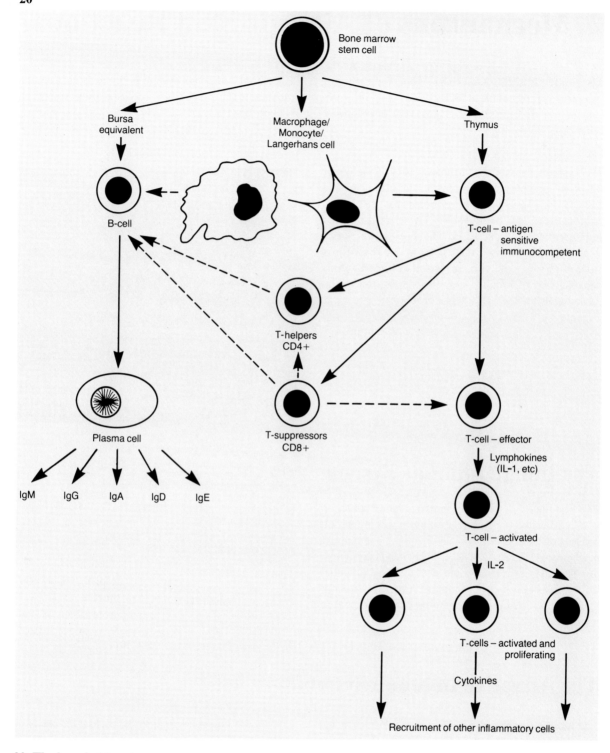

20 The lymphoid system.

Adaptive immunity is mediated by the lymphoid system (**20**). This system can respond to a variety of antigenic foreign material, irrespective of whether the material is potentially harmful or not. It produces two major populations of immunocompetent cells – thymus-dependent or T-cells and bursa-dependent or B-cells. These effect, respectively, cell-mediated and antibody-mediated specific immunity.

The humoral immune response

Antibodies are produced by B-cells in response to an antigenic stimulus, but this process requires the involvement of macrophages and helper T-cells. T-cell populations modulate both the cellular and humoral immune responses through a complex set of subpopulations of suppressor, helper, and activated T-lymphocytes. The products of the B-cells, antibodies, are found in five classes: IgM, IgG, IgA, IgD, and IgE. Each has a broadly similar, but unique, structure and funtion (**21** and *Table 5*).

Table 5. *Comparison of human immunoglobulin classes.*

Immuno-globin Class	Serum Concentration (Adult)	Half-life (Days)	Role
IgG	9.5–16.5 g/l	18–23	Precipitins, antitoxins
IgA	0.9–4.5 g/l	5–6.5	Surface protection
IgM	0.6–2.0 g/l	5	Agglutinins, opsonins, lysins, earliest antibody
IgD	3.0–400 mg/l	2–8	On lymphocyte surface of newborn
IgE	10.0–130 mg/l	2.3	Involved in atopy. Raised in parasitic infections

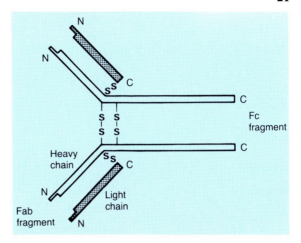

21 The basic structure of immunoglobulins. Each immunoglobin molecule consists of two identical light polypeptide chains and two heavy polypeptide chains, linked together by disulphide bonds (S–S). Note the position of the amino (N) and carboxyl (C) terminal ends of the peptide chains. The amino terminal ends are the antigen binding sites, hence this end of the molecule is known as the Fab fragment. The Fc fragment has sites for complement fixation, reactivity with rheumatoid factors, membrane transmission, macrophage fixation, and regulation of catabolism.

The cellular immune response

The products of the cellular immune response, antigen-sensitised lymphocytes, are composed of several subpopulations of T-cells, with varying physicochemical, antigenic, and functional characteristics. Upon encountering antigens, the immune system may variably activate a number of effector systems, including the mediators from basophil granules, complement, prostaglandins, kinins, and lymphokines. These stimulate the body's specific and non-specific defence mechanisms of inflammation. At the same time, the response creates a reserve of 'memory cells' for future demands.

The Skin Immune System

The epidermis contains highly specialised antigen-presenting cells called Langerhans cells (**20, 22**). These process antigen and present it to appropriate T-helper lymphocytes, inducing cytokine release, T-cell proliferation, and inflammation. Keratinocytes also secrete cytokines (**21**) which aid this response.

Both processes (induction) give rise to a clone of lymphocytes which are sensitised to a particular antigen; i.e. which specifically recognise that antigen. Subsequent challenge with the antigen produces cutaneous inflammatory responses.

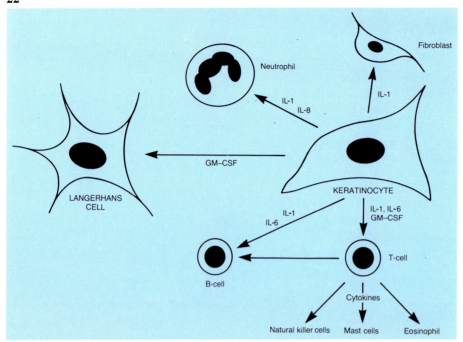

22 The keratinocyte cytokine cascade: the specialised skin immune system (IL = interleukin; GM–CSF = granulocyte-macrophage colony stimulating factor).

Abnormalities of the Immune System

A failure of any part of the immune system may predispose to infection, malignancy, or allergy. A depressed immune response is not always easy to diagnose clinically, and may be secondary to a number of causes, including HIV infection.

Apparently immune responses are not always triggered by sensitisation to antigens. For example, so-called pseudo-allergic reactions may occur in response to various drugs, and these may cause anaphylaxis, haemolytic anaemia, immune complex disease, and delayed cell-mediated responses in non-sensitised individuals. The mechanisms involve direct effects on prostaglandin release, mast cell, or complement activity.

In addition, non-specific tissue mechanisms of inflammation can be triggered by immune reactions which become amplified to produce clinical features identical to immunologically mediated diseases. The bronchial response to histamine, for example, may often be a combined effect of tissue reactivity and allergy in asthmatics. Similar combinations probably account for the generalised hyper-reactivity which is seen in the skin of some patients with atopic eczema and other allergic skin diseases.

Hypersensitivity reactions

Deleterious or inappropriate immune responses are termed hypersensitivity reactions. The Gell and Coombs classification (see *Table 3*) divides these reactions into four types, according to their immunopathological mechanisms, but in many, if not most, clinical situations more than one immunological mechanism may be involved. In atopic eczema, for example, Type I and Type IV reactions both play an important role.

Classification of hypersensitivity reactions

The mechanisms of Gell and Coombs reactions of Types I–IV are summarised in **23**, and their involvement in skin disorders is reviewed in *Table 6*.

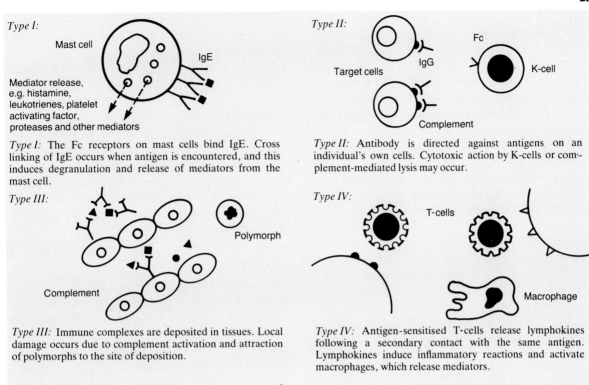

23 The mechanisms involved in hypersensitivity reactions (classified as by Gell and Coombs into Types I–IV).

Table 6. *Gell and Coombs' types of mechanisms of skin injury.*

Immune type	I	II	III	IV
Alternative name	Immediate	Cytotoxic antibody	Antigen–antibody immune-complex	Delayed-type Cell-mediated
Cells involved	Mast cell Basophil Eosinophil	B- or K-lymphocyte Macrophage	B-lymphocyte Polymorph Platelets	T-lymphocyte Macrophage Giant and epithelioid
Immunoglobulin	IgE	IgE; IgM	IgG	–
Skin disorder	Urticaria Angioedema Atopic eczema (early stages)	Pemphigus Pemphigoid Dermatitis herpetiformis Lupus erythematosus Scleroderma Dermatomyositis Relapsing polychondritis	Leucocytoclastic vasculitis Livedo vasculitis Polyarteritis nodosa Erythema nodosum Erythema multiforme Rheumatoid vasculitis Temporal arteritis Granulomatous vasculitis	Contact dermatitis Photo-allergic dermatitis Atopic eczema (late stages) Erythema multiforme? Patch tests Lymphocyte transformation
Appropriate investigations	Skin prick tests Specific serum IgE (RAST)	Immunofluorescence	Circulating immune complexes Complement conversion High ESR Immunofluorescence	Macrophage migration inhibition Cell-mediated cytotoxicity

Type I

This type of response is triggered by antigen which has penetrated body surfaces, for example skin, respiratory, or gastrointestinal tract. The antigen combines with cell-bound (reaginic) antibody on mast or basophil cell membranes. Bridging of IgE molecules on the mast cell surface triggers an immediate local release of vasoactive amines, initiated by a fall in cellular cyclic AMP. This response is normally transient and limited by the influence of suppressor T-cells. When IgE antibody reaches higher levels this response can lead to urticaria or asthma, due to the release of histamine and other mediators. In the extreme case, this mediator release can lead to acute anaphylaxis, which is potentially fatal (for example, following penicillin injection or an insect sting in a sensitised patient).

Atopic patients have a familial tendency to develop abnormal hypersensitivity to common allergens. The atopic trait may be defined as the spontaneous tendency of an individual to produce high levels of IgE antibodies against one or more common antigens, in association with antigen-provoked disorders in which reaginic mechanisms can be identified. Examples include extrinsic allergic asthma, allergic rhinitis, allergic conjunctivitis, urticaria, and atopic-eczema.

Type II

This response is initiated by antibody reacting with antigenic components of cell or tissue elements. Complement fixation and/or K-cell lysis lead to damage. The classic example is the reaction which follows an incompatible blood transfusion. Some drugs can adsorb onto cell membranes and then immunologically cause haemolysis, agranulocytosis, or thrombocytopenia. A similar clincal effect may be produced by low concentrations of lympho-cytotoxins, as in systemic lupus erythematosus (SLE). Antireceptor antibody can also have a blocking effect, as in myasthenia gravis.

Occasionally, antibodies bind to the suface of a cell without causing its death or activating complement. Instead, the cell is stimulated to produce a hormone-like substance which may mediate disease, as in pemphigus.

Type III

This response occurs when antigen reacts in tissue spaces with potentially precipitating antibody, forming microprecipitates in and around small blood vessels, and causing secondary damage to cells. When antigen is in excess, soluble circulating immune complexes are formed and deposited in the endothelial lining of blood vessel walls or the basement membrane, fixing complement and causing local inflammation. This inflammation may be acute, as in serum sickness, with fever, vasculitis, skin rash, proteinuria, and joint inflammation; or it may be chronic, as in SLE, uveitis, vasculitis, or glomerulonephritis.

Type IV

Several different types of immune reaction can produce delayed hypersensitivity. Unlike other types of hypersensitivity, they cannot be transferred from one individual to another by serum, but can be transferred by certain T-lymphocytes. The Type IV reaction involves active sensitised T-lymphocytes, which respond specifically to allergen by the release of lymphokines and/or the development of cytotoxicity. Locally, the Type IV reaction is manifested by the infiltration of cells at the site of antigen injection. Lymphokines are responsible for the recruitment of lymphocytes and the activation of local macrophages. Cells are identified as targets for cell-mediated immune attack by surface antigenic determinants which are immunogenic in the host. These may be histocompatibility antigens, new membrane antigens induced by viral, bacterial, or other infection, tumour-specific antigens, or native surface antigens involved in autoimmune reactions.

Cell-mediated immune reactions are common in the defence against fungal and viral infections of the skin. They are also important in granulomatous reactions, delayed hypersensitivity reactions and allergic contact dermatitis. They probably play a role in some photosensitive disorders, in protecting against carcinogenesis and in mediating reactions to insect bites.

3 Investigation of Skin Allergy

In skin disease, the patient's history and the findings on examination provide valuable clues to the probable underlying diagnosis, as outlined in Chapter 1. Often, a presumptive diagnosis will be possible on the basis of the history and examination alone, but further investigations may be needed to confirm the diagnosis or to investigate its underlying cause.

Where the patient describes episodes of urticaria or angioedema, physical signs may be completely absent at the time of consultation. Diagnosis can sometimes be aided in these circumstances by examining photographs taken by the patient's friends or relatives during an attack (**24**). A formal test for dermographism during the examination of the patient (**25**) may also provide evidence of an urticarial tendency (though not of a definite immunological mechanism).

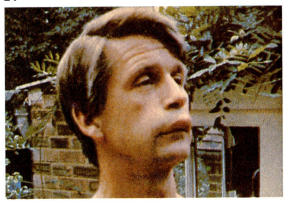

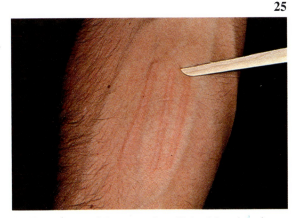

24 Family photographs can be of value in the diagnosis of a transient condition such as angioedema. The patient's wife took this photograph during one of his first attacks of angioedema, and it was helpful in confirming the diagnosis when he attended the clinic. One attack occurred after he had taken aspirin, but he continued to suffer from recurrent attacks despite avoiding the drug. These resulted from his sensitivity to salicylates in natural and processed foods. An exclusion diet confirmed the diagnosis and prevented all but the occasional attack (see Chapter 9).

25 Dermographism can be elicited by drawing a broken tongue depressor over the skin of the forearm or back. A positive test is one which produces a weal 2 mm or more in width within about 1–3 minutes, and the test usually elicits an exaggerated triple response. A red line occurs within a few seconds, due to capillary dilatation. This is followed by a broadening area of erythema (the axon-reflex flare, from arteriolar dilatation). The red line is then replaced by a weal with surrounding erythema; this results from transudation of fluid through the dilated capillaries. As a control, the physician can perform this test on his own arm at the same time (unless, of course, he or she also has dermographism).

Patch Tests

Patch tests are a valuable tool in the diagnosis of allergic contact dermatitis and in establishing its cause. They should usually be carried out when a patient presents with eczematous lesions of the hands, feet, or face – common sites for allergic contact dermatitis; and they should also be used when contact dermatitis is suspected elsewhere on the body. They should not be used for patients with severe acute eczema, as the results may be misleading at this stage.

The allergens are formulated in appropriate concentrations and placed in shallow aluminium wells of about 1 cm^2 known as Finn chambers (**26, 27**). The wells are applied in strips to the patient's

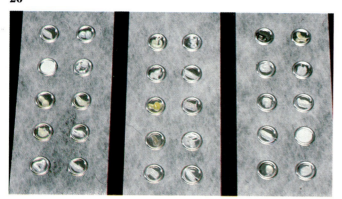

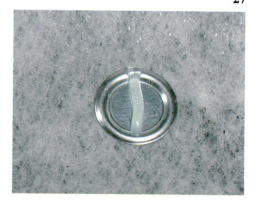

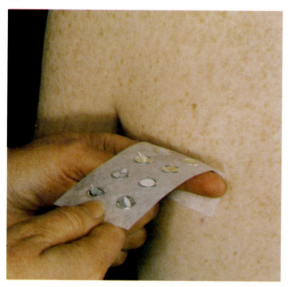

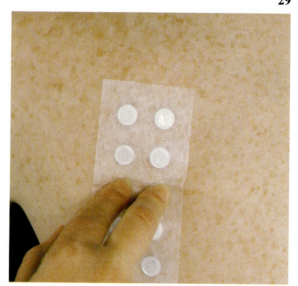

26–30 The patch testing procedure uses pre-assembled aluminium chambers (Finn chambers), which are placed in strips on hypo-allergenic tape and prepared for application to the patient's back. The upper back is the preferred test site, but if the back is eczematous, another skin area may be used. Allergens in solution form are applied, using a pipette or orange stick, to filter discs which are placed within the chambers. Two are shown in **26**. Most allergens are diluted in petrolatum, and these are applied in a line across the diameter of the chamber. No special skin preparation is required. The chambers are fixed to the back from the bottom upwards (**28**) and then pressed firmly against the skin to expel air and spread the allergen evenly over the area occluded by the chamber (**29**). Several strips may be applied. The sites of application should be carefully labelled by marking the patient's skin with a pen (**30**) and, obviously, the location of each allergen must be carefully recorded on an appropriate record sheet.

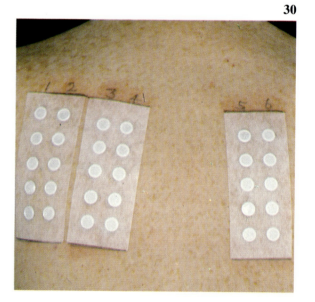

back and kept in place by hypo-allergenic tape (**28–30**). The skin is marked appropriately, and the patient asked to keep the area dry.

The patches are removed after 48 hours and the skin examined for a positive response, characterised by itching and erythematous swelling, and often accompanied by vesication; all of these may extend beyond the margin of the patch when responses are strongly positive. With most substances the allergic response is maximal at 48 h, but some chemicals (e.g. neomycin) cause a later response, so a second reading of the patches at 96 h is routine, and later responses should be reported by the patient. Patch test reactions are graded at each reading (*Table 7* and **31–33**).

Table 7. *Patch test reading and interpretation.*

The test reactions are graded at each reading as follows:	
+	Weak (non-vesicular) positive reaction: erythema, infiltration, possibly papules.
++	Strong (oedematous or vesicular) positive reaction (**24**).
+++	Extreme (spreading, bullous, ulcerative) positive reaction (**25**).
–	Negative reaction.
IR	Irritant reactions.
NT	Not tested.

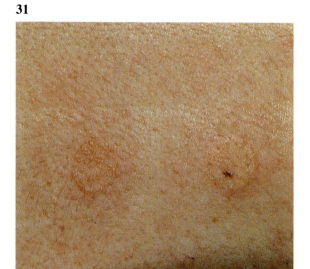
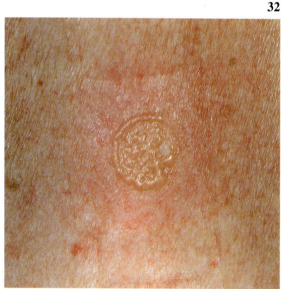

31, 32 Typical positive patch test results, as commonly seen at 48 hours. The two results in **31** are both ++, showing erythema and vesicle formation. The result in **32** is +++ (extreme) with extensive vesication and bullae. Ulceration may well occur on this site at a later stage.

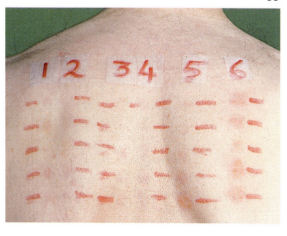

33 Multiple positive patch tests in a gardener who seemed to have become sensitised to chrysanthemums. Extracts from various chrysanthemum plants were specially prepared, and the test results confirmed that he was sensitive to all the chrysanthemum types which he grew. Some cross-sensitivity to other *Compositae* plants was also demonstrated.

Patch testing is simple and clinically useful, but the results are not always easy to interpret. The classic reaction is due to a cell-mediated delayed hypersensitivity (Type IV) response, but false positive reactions may occur. A common cause of false positive reactions is the 'angry back' or 'excited skin' syndrome. This may occur in up to 40% of patients with multiple positive reactions. It is a phenomenon in which a very strong result (+++) produces a state of skin hyper-reactivity, causing other patch test sites to become reactive with a questionable or + reaction. Another cause of false positive reactions is the use of irritant chemicals for patch testing. This is generally avoided when a standard battery of allergens obtained from commercial sources is used.

The formulation of the allergens is critical and various standard contact allergen batteries have been developed in different areas of the world to include most of the common allergens in contact dermatitis (e.g. *Table 8*). These include metallic ions, rubber accelerators and antioxidants, topical drugs, and other sensitising substances. The composition of these batteries varies from place to place and from time to time.

Table 8. *Some common allergens in contact dermatitis.*

Allergen	Sources
Nickel	Jewellery, jean studs, bra clips, tools
Balsam of Peru	Perfumes, citrus fruits
Dichromate	Cement, leather, matches
Paraphenylenediamine	Hair dyes, clothing
Rubber chemicals	Shoes, clothing, gloves
Colophony (rosin)	Sticking plaster, collodium
Neomycin	Topical medicaments
Benzocaine	Topical anaesthetics
Parabens	Preservatives in cosmetics and creams
Wool alcohols	Lanolin, cosmetics, creams
Imidazolidinyl urea	Preservative in creams and cosmetics
Formaldehyde (aqueous)	Clothing, cosmetics, glues, paper
Epoxy resin	Glues

Other forms of patch testing

Some substances are too irritant to apply constantly in a standard patch test. They may be tested by simple repetitive contact over several days – usually on the skin of the volar surface of the forearm.

A recent development in this form of contact testing has been the use of house dust mite extracts. Many patients with atopic eczema show a positive reaction to dust mite extracts on contact testing. The relevance of this finding is not yet completely clear, but it supports the view that dust mite allergy may play a role in some patients with atopic eczema (see Chapter 7). The test is not yet applicable as a routine procedure.

In patients with urticaria, contact testing with suspected allergens is occasionally useful (see Chapter 4). The test substance is applied to the volar surface of the forearm without any form of prick or scratch. The test is positive if an urticarial response develops within 20–30 minutes.

Photopatch testing

Photopatch testing is useful in the investigation of possible phototoxic or photoallergic reactions (see Chapters 7 and 8). In these conditions, a skin reaction occurs when an area exposed to a potentially allergenic or toxic substance is subsequently exposed to light. This reaction is mimicked in the test, where a special ultraviolet light source, similar to that used in PUVA treatment, is used to light the skin after potential photosensitisers have been applied (**34**).

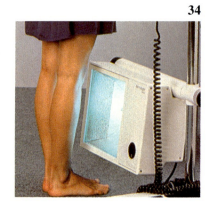

34

34 Photopatch testing may be carried out using the kind of light source normally used for PUVA treatment. Here, the ultraviolet light source is being used to treat local areas of psoriasis on the legs. For photopatch testing the suspected allergens would be applied to the back and exposed in the same way.

Skin Prick Tests

Skin prick tests often provide useful confirmatory evidence of reaction to suspected allergens in respiratory conditions, but they have a lesser role in allergic skin disease. The technique is simple, and with standardised allergen solutions it gives reproducible results (**35, 36**). Isolated positive results are good evidence of a Type I allergic response. Late reactions may also occur after 24–48 hours, and these represent delayed (Type IV) hypersensitivity to the allergen.

Dermographism may lead to false positive results, while antihistamine treatment may cause false negative results. Both possibilities can be excluded by including saline and histamine controls in the test battery. More confusing are the multiple positive results found in some patients with severe atopic eczema. The clinical relevance of these is unclear, but they do not necessarily signify multiple Type I allergies, and they are not helpful in management.

Prick tests may occasionally be helpful in tracking down the cause of non-dermographic urticaria – though the allergen will usually have been suspected from the history, and the history is always more important than the test result. Apart from this, prick tests have little value in allergic skin disorders.

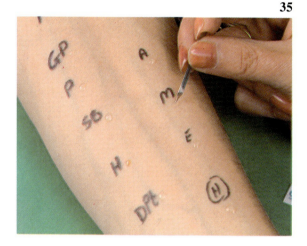

35 In skin prick testing, the skin is cleaned, prick sites are marked, and a small drop of each allergen solution is placed on the skin. A lance is introduced through the drop to a depth of about 1 mm into the skin and pulled out, raising the skin in the process – the skin should not bleed – and the site is blotted dry. The lance can be wiped throroughly dry with a sterile swab and re-used with another solution on the same patient.

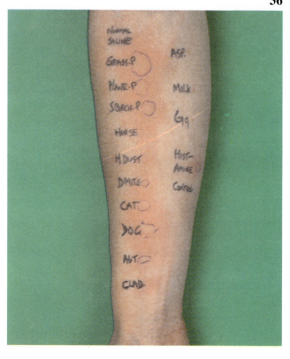

36 A multiple positive prick test result. This patient had mild atopic eczema. His symptoms of hay fever from April to August correlate with the positive reactions to grass, and to plane and silver birch pollens. He also developed nasal and eye symptoms on contact with cats – but despite the positive skin test, dogs did not cause obvious symptoms, and there was nothing to suggest that *Alternaria* contributed to his rhinitis. Note that the other allergens gave negative results – the flare reactions should be regarded as non-specific, as there was no measurable weal. Although of some value in assessing the patient's nasal and eye symptoms, these results do not provide any useful information on the cause or management of his eczema.

Skin Biopsy

Skin biopsy is an important technique in the definitive diagnosis of many allergic skin disorders. Samples may be obtained by ellipse excision (**37**) or by punch biopsy (**38**), and examined histologically (**39**) and by direct immunoflourescence techniques (**40**). In blistering diseases, biopsy of the perilesional skin is usually necessary to establish the level of the split and the level at which immunoglobulins are deposited.

37

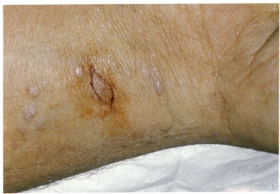

38

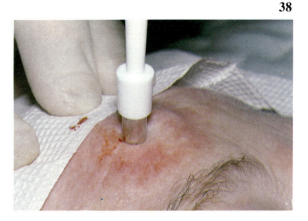

37 Ellipse excision biopsy is a more complex procedure than punch biopsy (**38**) and the wound usually requires suturing. Healing is rapid, however, and if the incision is made in the line of a skin crease no significant scar need result.

38 Punch biopsy is a very simple technique. The area to be biopsied is limited by the area of the punch, and a scalpel is still necessary to remove the punched-out area of skin. Suturing is not always necessary, but healing by primary intention (without suturing) may take several weeks, although significant scarring is unusual.

39

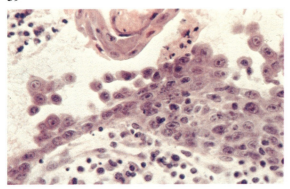

40

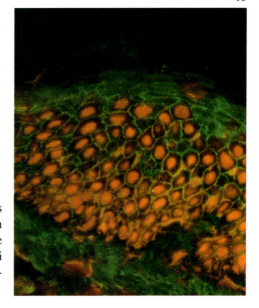

39 A high power view of the epidermis and superficial dermis from a routine biopsy in a patient with pemphigus vulgaris. Note the disintegration of the epidermis with rounding of the keratinocytes. The resulting blister is supra-basal. The blistering is associated with intense dermal inflammation.

40 Direct immunofluorescence on a skin biopsy. This biopsy was taken from a perilesional area in a patient with pemphigus vulgaris. Note the intercellular positive immunofluoresence staining due to bound IgG. The nuclei of the keratinocytes within the epidermis are counter-stained orange–red to ease interpretation of this specimen.

Investigations on Peripheral Blood

A number of investigations on peripheral blood may be useful in some patients with allergic skin disease (**41**).

Serum immunoglobulins

Serum immunoglobulin levels can be measured, but this is rarely helpful in the management of allergic skin disease. In atopic individuals, the IgE level is often elevated, and the IgA level is occasionally depressed, but Type I allergic responses can occur with a normal serum IgE level. A consistent grossly elevated IgE level is often associated with intestinal parasitic infestation, and should not be attributed to atopy alone without further investigation.

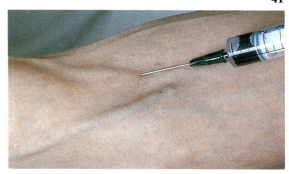

41 Venous blood sampling is required for a number of useful investigations in allergic skin disease. The nature of the tests carried out will depend upon the clinical problem (see text).

The radioallergosorbent test (RAST)

The concentration of circulating IgE is very low and it is not possible to measure the level of IgE antibodies to specific antigens directly. This can be overcome by the RAST method (**42**).

In general, the RAST method produces results comparable with skin prick testing in Type I allergic disorders. It is an *in vitro* technique and the blood sample can be collected away from the laboratory; but it does not provide immediate information and it is expensive. In addition, a theoretical objection is that IgE RASTs cannot detect IgG-mediated reactions, which may conceivably be detected on skin testing. The extent of use of the RAST method varies from one centre to another, but – as with skin prick testing – its role in assessing allergic skin disorders is relatively small.

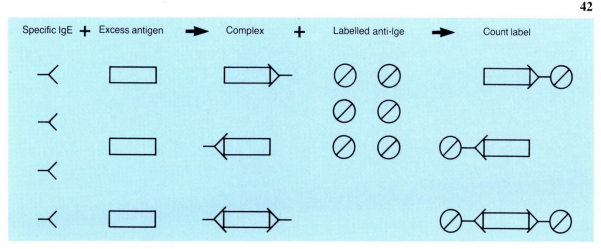

42 The radioallergosorbent test (RAST) method. The antigen under test is bound to insoluble particles (usually on a cellulose disc), and these are incubated with the patient's serum. IgE antibodies to the antigen in the serum will bind to the sensitised particles, forming a complex. A radioactively labelled antiserum to IgE is added, the insoluble particles are separated (the disc is washed), and their radioactivity assessed. The resulting 'RAST score' varies directly in proportion with the concentration of specific IgE in the patient's serum.

Autoantibodies

The identification of autoantibodies is an important step in the diagnosis of connective tissue diseases with dermatological manifestations. Autoantibodies to various organelles and tissues may be found in the serum. Many can be identified by indirect immunofluorescence and, in some bullous disorders, autoantibody titres correlate with disease severity and are useful in long-term monitoring. Cryostat sections of appropriate human or animal tissue containing the relevant antigens are incubated with the patient's serum. A fluorescein-labelled reagent is then added, revealing the sites at which immunoglobulin has become bound to the tissue section (**43, 44**). A number of other techniques, including radio-immunoassay and agglutination may also be used to identify autoantibodies.

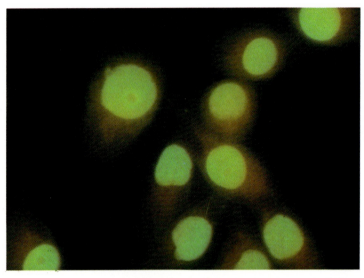

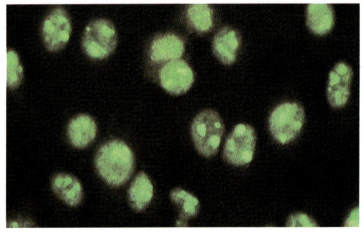

43, 44 Indirect immunofluorescence tests that were performed on human cell lines using serum from patients with dermatological manifestations suggesting connective tissue disorders. Both tests show antinuclear antibodies. **43** shows a homogenous pattern, consistent with the diagnosis of systemic lupus erythematosus. **44** shows a nucleolar pattern; this pattern is usually found in patients with systemic sclerosis.

Lupus erythematosus (LE) cells

In 90% of patients with systemic lupus erythematosus (SLE), LE cells can be found in the peripheral blood (**45**).

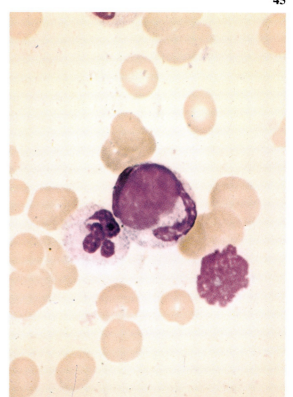

45 A lupus erythematosus cell (LE cell). The LE cell is a polymorphonuclear leucocyte (a neutrophil) in which characteristic inclusions of nuclear material are found within the cytoplasm after the blood has been left standing. The appearances of these cells may vary, but they will be recognised by a skilled microscopist. LE cells are found in the blood of 90% of patients with systemic lupus erythematosus (SLE).

Eosinophilia

An eosinophil count of more than 4% of the total white cells may occur in atopic subjects (**46**), though massive eosinophilia is unusual and requires investigation, e.g. for intestinal parasites.

46 A normal eosinophil polymorph, showing the characteristic 'spectacle' arrangement of the nuclear segments, which are usually two in number. An eosinophil count of more than 4% of the total white cells may occur in atopic subjects, though other causes such as intestinal parasites must be excluded if the eosinophil count is very high.

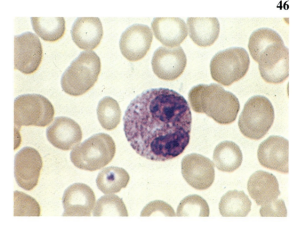

Other blood tests

These may be valuable in specific circumstances, in order to investigate the systemic consequences of allergic disorders with skin manifestations, or to assess the underlying immunological abnormalities in greater detail.

Other investigations

Exclusion diets may be helpful in the diagnosis of skin disease associated with food intolerance (see Chapter 9).

It is important to remember that allergic skin disease may be associated with disorders of other systems. Patients with atopic eczema often have associated allergic rhinitis, conjunctivitis, and asthma; and the asthma frequently remains undiagnosed, especially in childhood. Peak flow measurement (**47**) is simple and should be carried out (repeatedly, if necessary) in any atopic child with any form of respiratory symptoms.

Patients with dermatitis herpetiformis usually have villous atrophy and a flattened small bowel mucosa. Investigation by jejunal biopsy and the assessment of possible malabsorption should be routine in such patients.

Multisystem immunological disorders, such as SLE and rheumatoid arthritis, will often need extensive investigation beyond the skin, to assess and monitor damage to other organ systems.

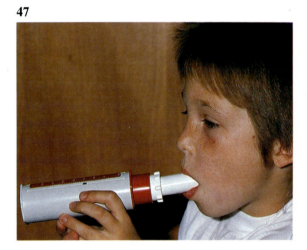

47 Wheezing or other respiratory symptoms in children with atopic eczema are commonly due to undiagnosed asthma. Peak expiratory flow measurement is a simple method of investigating and monitoring these patients. It is always important to remember the possible involvement of other organ systems in allergic skin disease.

4 Skin Disorders Associated with Immediate Allergic Reactions

Urticaria

Urticaria is a common reaction pattern in the skin and is not a disease entity in its own right. When allergic in origin, it is the classic example of an immediate (Gell and Coombs Type I) reaction. The characteristic weals (hives) of this condition are due to vasodilation and leakage of fluid into the dermis (**48–50**).

Individual weals are transient, usually lasting for just a few hours before resolving spontaneously, but lesions may recur subsequently at either the same or different sites. Urticaria may be *acute,* in which case lesions cease to appear within 6 weeks of onset, or *chronic,* where lesions recur for more than 6 weeks.

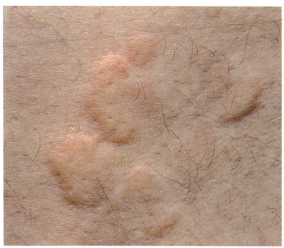

48 Urticaria may be acute or chronic and results from localised vasodilatation and the transudation of fluid from the small blood vessels in the upper dermis. Several chemical mediators may be involved, including histamine. Mediator release is sometimes caused by IgE-mediated hypersensitivity (Type I). The characteristic lesions are transient, pruritic, erythematous weals (hives). Individual urticarial lesions usually disappear without trace within 24 hours of onset. Persistence of lesions or residual bruising, especially if associated with systemic symptoms, should alert the clinician to the possibility of urticarial vasculitis.

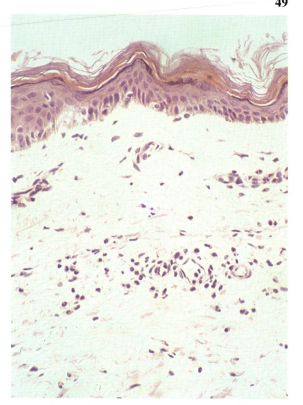

49 Urticaria has a characteristic histopathological appearance, though skin biopsy is not routinely required for diagnosis. There is a mild, loosely textured, upper dermal mixed inflammatory infiltrate around dilated upper dermal blood vessels. Vasculitis is not a feature. The surrounding dermis is often oedematous.

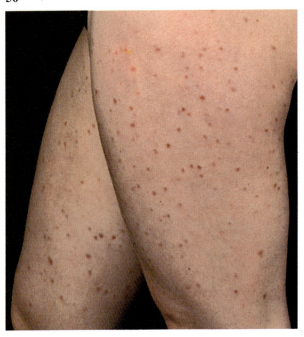

50 Urticaria pigmentosa (mastocytosis) is a condition in which there is dermal accumulation of mast cells. It presents as brownish macules in the skin, which urticate on friction, due to the direct release of mediators. It is not an allergic condition. Childhood and adult forms are recognised, and both can be associated with systemic mastocytosis.

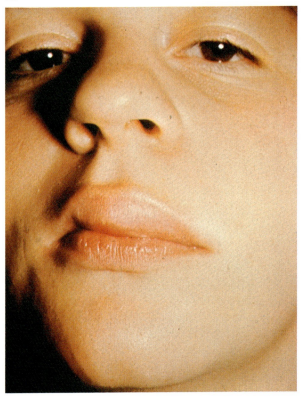

51 Urticaria affecting the lips and face is often referred to as angioedema. This patient's angioedema is largely confined to the lips, especially the upper lip. The ususal cause of angioedema of the lips is hypersensitivity or allergy to food, such as shellfish or peanuts (see Chapter 9). In these circumstances, urticaria may be absent from the rest of the body, but there is a risk of gastrointestinal or respiratory involvement.

Angioedema is a term used to describe urticaria affecting the face and lips (**51–53**). The oedema commonly extends into the subcutaneous tissues, and in severe cases there may be life-threatening oedema of the larynx (**54**), and oedematous involvement of the lower respiratory tract, gut, or joints.

Urticaria and angioedema are common: 15–20% of the population experience at least one episode during their lifetime. When urticaria is acute, the cause can usually be found. In patients with chronic urticaria the cause is found in only 25% of cases.

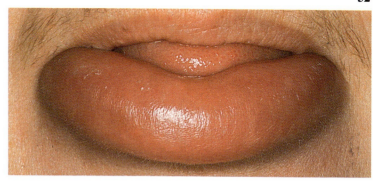

52 Angioedema affecting the lower lip. This patient had a long history of painless, itchy, transient swelling of the lips and face, and there was no clinical suggestion of sensitivity to particular foods. Further investigations revealed a diminished serum C_1-esterase inhibitor level. The underlying cause here is hereditary angioedema – not an allergic condition.

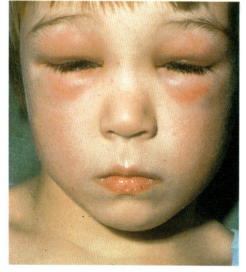

53 Angioedema affecting the face, and especially the periorbital skin. In this 4-year-old boy, the condition presented acutely, following a wasp sting. The immediate discomfort and impairment of vision may be relieved by systemic antihistamine therapy and the local application of ice packs, but it is important to bear in mind the possibility of laryngeal oedema or an anaphylactic reaction. Intravenous hydrocortisone or even adrenaline may be required in these circumstances.

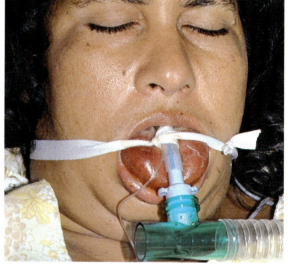

54 Severe angioedema in this 43-year-old woman was accompanied by laryngeal obstruction and she required urgent life-saving endotracheal intubation. Note the oedema of her face, mouth, and tongue. This case provides an important reminder that severe angioedema can be a fatal condition.

Table 9. *Classification of urticaria.*

	Aetiology
Immunological	
IgE dependent	Atopic Specific antigen sensitivity, e.g. food, worms
Physical	Dermographism, pressure, heat, water, cold, sunlight, cholinergic, etc. (see *Table 11*)
Complement-mediated	Hereditary angioedema, e.g. C-esterase inhibitor deficiency Acquired, e.g. lymphoma Autoimmune
Non-immunological	
Substances which directly stimulate mast cell degranulation	Drugs, e.g. opiates, quinine, chlortetracycline, aspirin Chemicals, e.g. dextran, azo-dyes, benzoates Food, e.g. egg white, strawberries, and shellfish
Histamine-containing foods	e.g. some cheeses, mackerel, and tuna fish
Physical agents and cholinergic effects	
Contact urticaria	

Table 10. *Provoking factors in urticaria.*

Exogenous factors
Food and food additives (e.g. shellfish, tartrazine)
Drugs (topical and systemic)
Insect bites
Pollen
Inhalants
Animal dander
Physical stimuli

Endogenous factors
Intestinal parasites
Connective tissue disorder, e.g. lupus erythematosus
Autoimmune thyroid disease
Diabetes
Cancer/lymphoma
Pregnancy

Both immunological and non-immunological factors may precipitate urticaria (see *Table 9*). Although Type I allergy is an important cause, non-allergic mechanisms are more common. Non-allergic urticaria or angioedema may occur on first exposure to a provoking substance or event, whereas IgE-mediated urticaria requires sensitisation from prior exposure to the provoking agent or a related substance. Provoking factors in urticaria may be exogenous or endogenous (*Table 10*).

Types of urticaria

IgE-dependent (hypersensitivity) urticaria

This is due to a class IgE (and sometimes IgG4) mediated (Type I) allergic reaction (see Chaper 2). Allergens may be encountered by ingestion of food, by inhalation, by injection, from parasites, from infections, or from insect bites.

Chronic idiopathic urticaria

This type of urticaria is very common, accounting for about three quarters of patients who present with this symptom. The majority of patients who develop prolonged, continuous, or frequently repeated episodes of urticaria are not atopic and they have normal IgE concentrations.

The onset is usually fairly abrupt and no precipitating causes are apparent; fortunately, most cases resolve spontaneously within 2 years, but symptoms may persist for 10 years or more in about 20% of patients. Abnormalities of complement factors have been demonstrated in some patients, mainly in so-called urticarial vasculitis (see Chapter 6).

Physical urticaria

A large number of variants of urticaria which are provoked by physical stimuli have been described.

Their major characteristics are summarised in *Table 11*.

Table 11. Comparison of the physical urticarias.

Urticaria	Relative frequency	Precipitant	Time of onset	Duration	Local symptoms	Systemic symptoms	Tests	Mechanism	Treatment
Symptomatic dermographism	Most frequent	Stroking skin	Minutes	2–3 hours	Irregular, pruritic weals	None	Scratch skin	Passive transfer; IgE; histamine; possible role of adenosine triphosphate; substance P; posssible direct pharmacological mechanism	Continuous antihistamine regimen; combined H_1 and H_2 blockers
Delayed pressure urticaria	Frequent	Pressure	3–12 hours	8–24 hours	Diffuse tender swelling	Flu-like symptoms	Apply weight	Unknown	Avoidance of precipitants; if severe, antihistamines or low dosages of corticosteroids given for systemic effect
Solar urticaria	Uncommon	Various wavelengths of light	2–5 minutes	15 minutes –3 hours	Pruritic weals	Wheezing; dizziness; syncope	Phototest	Passive transfer; reverse passive transfer; IgE; possibly histamine	Avoidance of precipitants; antihistamines; sunscreens; chloroquine phosphate regimen for short time
Cold urticaria	Frequent	Cold contact	2–5 minutes	1–2 hours	Pruritic weals	Wheezing; syncope; drowning	Apply ice-filled copper beaker to arm; immerse in cold water	Passive transfer; reverse passive transfer; IgE (IgM); histamine vasculitis can be induced	Antihistamines; desensitisation; avoidance of precipitants
Heat urticaria	Rare	Heat contact	2–5 minutes rarely delayed	1 hour	Pruritic weals	None	Apply hot water filled cylinder to arm	Possibly histamine; possibly complement	Antihistamines; desensitisation; avoidance of precipitants
Cholinergic urticaria	Very frequent	General overheating of body, exercise, stress	2–20 minutes	30 minutes – 1 hour	Papular, pruritic weals	Syncope; diarrhoea vomiting; salivation; headaches	Bathe in hot water; exercise until perspiring; inject methacholine chloride	Passive transfer; possibly immunoglobulin; product of sweat gland stimulation; histamine; reduced protease inhibitor	Application of cold water or ice to skin; antihistamines; refractory period; anticholinergics
Aquagenic urticaria	Rare	Water contact	Several minutes to 30 minutes	30–45 minutes	Papular, pruritic weals	None reported	Apply water compresses to skin	Unknown	Avoidance of precipitants; antihistamines; application of inert oil
Vibratory angioedema	Very rare	Vibrating against skin	2–5 minutes	1 hour	Angioedema	None reported	Apply body of vibrating mixer to forearm	Unknown	Avoidance of precipitants

Modified from Jorizzo JL and Smith EB: *Arch. Dermatol.* **118**: 198, 1982.

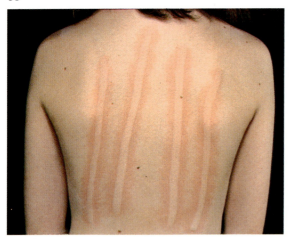

Dermographism

In this common form of urticaria (**9, 55**), mast cells in the skin release histamine after rubbing or scratching. The linear weals are therefore an exaggerated triple response of Lewis, which can be elicited as a physical sign (**25**).

55 Dermographism is the most common form of physical urticaria. It may be hereditary or acquired. A linear weal and flare reaction develops within 2–3 minutes of scratching normal skin with a blunt instrument or fingernail. The sign can be easily confirmed by the clinician, using an orange stick or or tongue depressor (**25**). Antihistamine treatment is usually effective and undue trauma to the skin should be avoided.

Delayed pressure urticaria

This type of urticaria develops after 3–6 hours and can last 48 hours. As the name suggests, it occurs particularly on the feet, hands and buttocks. It is probably mediated by kinins and prostaglandins, rather than by histamine.

Temperature-dependent urticaria

These types of urticaria can be reproduced in the clinic by exposing the skin to extremes of temperature. Urticaria may be provoked by heat or by cold (**56**). Occasionally, cold urticaria is the presenting feature of cryoglobulinaemia.

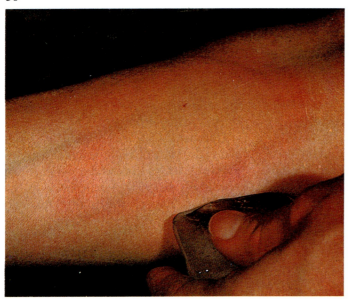

56 Cold urticaria developed in this patient within minutes of holding an ice cube against the skin; it lasted for several hours. The condition may be inherited as an autosomal dominant trait, but it is usually acquired, and there is no obvious reason for its onset. In severe cases, similar reactions may be provoked by cold air or water, and there may be oropharyngeal oedema on the ingestion of cold liquids. In very sensitive patients, reactions resembling anaphylactic shock may occur. Antihistamine treatment may be helpful.

Solar urticaria

This form of urticaria may be IgE-mediated, but some patients with solar urticaria have erythropoietic protoporphyria.

Cholinergic urticaria

Strenuous exercise, anxiety, or (sometimes) heat elicit this disorder. The eruption tends to be more papular than idiopathic urticaria (**57**). It is mediated by acetylcholine which is released from parasympathetic nerves in the skin and which causes vasodilatation.

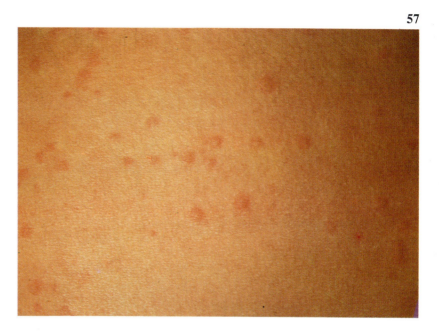

57 Cholinergic urticaria is a distinctive type of urticaria in which small pruritic papules develop after stimuli, such as exercise, stress, and heat (e.g. taking a hot bath). The condition usually affects young adults, and appears on the upper trunk, but it may be more widespread. The lesions are characteristically very small and the episodes are short-lived, lasting 15–30 minutes. Itching is prominent and systemic symptoms, such as wheezing, rarely occur. Treatment with antihistamines may be helpful, and hydroxyzine hydrochloride – which also has a minor sedative action – may be particularly beneficial.

Contact urticaria

This type of urticaria may be IgE-mediated or may result from a pharmacological or idiopathic effect. Weals occur as a direct response to chemicals applied directly to the skin. A wide range of substances has been implicated (*Table 12*). Lesions occur within minutes to hours and resolve in less than 24 hours, leaving normal skin. There is a wide spectrum of clinical presentation in this group, ranging from minor symptoms to an anaphylactic response involving respiratory and gastrointestinal symptoms. Severe cases of contact urticaria may exhibit both immunological and non-immunological features, and these are of uncertain aetiology. The immunological component is a Type I, IgE-mediated hypersensitivity reaction, but IgM- and IgG-mediated activation of complement have also been implicated. The non-immunological component, in contrast to that in classical urticaria, is probably prostaglandin-mediated, as severe cases of non-immunological contact urticaria can sometimes be abolished by aspirin or indomethacin.

Table 12. *Substances implicated as causes of contact urticaria.*

Chemically defined	Chemically undefined	
Ammonium persulphate	Animals	Foods (*cont.*)
Bacitracin	Arthropod bites	Seafood
Balsam of Peru	Danders	Legumes
Benzoic acid	Marine organisms	Nuts
Chloramphenicol	Serum	Plants
Chlorpromazine	Saliva	Nettles
Epoxy resins	Cosmetics	Cactus
Formaldehyde	Nail varnish	Textiles
Lanolin	Hair spray	Wool
Para-aminodiphenylamine	Perfume	Silk
Parabens (ethyl- and methyl-)	Foods	Rubber
Penicillin	Chicken, eggs	Wood
Salicylic acid	Flour	Exotic woods
	Fruit	

Diagnosis and management of urticaria

Diagnosis is often self-evident, and in acute urticaria careful history taking often reveals an obvious cause. Where the diagnosis of urticaria is uncertain, a record of the patient's appearance during an attack may be helpful (**24**); and a test for dermographism (**25**) or other physical tests (*Table 11*) may be useful in revealing physical urticarias. Where a physical cause is discovered, further investigation is usually unnecessary.

Where individual lesions persist for more than 24 hours, or where lesions are painful, the possibility of urticarial vasculitis (Chapter 6) should be considered.

Contact urticaria may be further investigated by direct contact testing with suspected allergens or irritants (Chapter 3). Skin prick testing may also occasionally be useful where a Type I immunological response to particular antigens is suspected.

For patients with chronic urticaria, a detailed investigation for every possible underlying cause has been shown to be valueless. Where the cause is found, this is usually the result of clues identified by taking a thorough history and carrying out a full examination of the patient. Undiagnosed autoimmune thyroid disease is common enough to warrant routine thyroid function tests and autoantibody screening in obscure cases; and it is often sensible to undertake a trial of a relatively simple exclusion diet, especially one which excludes salicylates, azo-dyes, and benzoates (see Chapter 9). Other investigations may be carried out (*Table 13*), but are unlikely to be helpful in the absence of clinical clues.

In management, provoking substances and stimuli should be avoided wherever possible. It is essential to avoid mast cell degranulation caused by citric acid in fruit juice, or by drugs such as aspirin, non-steroidal anti-inflammatory drugs, and opiates. In idiopathic urticaria, when symptoms result from unavoidable causes, or when they persist despite control of the cause, antihistamines are the mainstay of treatment. Many of the trials of therapy, e.g. in the physical urticarias (*Table 11*), were carried out before the advent of non-sedating antihistamine therapy. The newer non-sedating antihistamines are now often very useful, but there is sometimes still a place for the use of a sedating antihistamine – especially at night when the lesions are pruritic. The addition of an H_2-receptor antagonist drug is sometimes helpful, especially in dermo-graphism where a combined H_1 and H_2 blockade has been shown to be more effective than an H_1 blockade alone.

In severe cases, there may be a role for tricyclic antidepressant drugs – especially doxepin, which also has potent antihistamine effects. Oral or injected corticosteroids, and even injected adrenaline, may be needed where life-threatening angioedema occurs.

Table 13. *Investigations which may be useful in some patients with chronic persistent urticaria.*

Full blood count and blood film
Erythrocyte sedimentation rate
Liver function tests
Chest X-ray, sinus X-rays
Examination of fresh stools for parasites
Examination of urine for bacteria
Complement screen, including C_1-esterase inhibitor
Autoantibodies (including thyroid)
Thyroid function tests
Exclusion diet
Hepatitis B surface antigen

Reactive Erythemas

Reactive erythema without urticaria may occur in response to many known or unknown stimuli and may take a number of different forms (*Table 14*). The mechanisms involved in some of these erythematous reactions are at least partially understood, and they usually involve Type III and/or Type IV hypersensitivity reactions. The mechanism behind erythema annulare (**58, 59**) is unclear, but it is thought to be a Type I response.

Table 14. *Some reactive erythemas.*

Erythema	Possible mechanism
Erythema annulare centrifugum	Type I
Erythema multiforme	Type III/Type IV
Erythema nodosum	Type III
Erythema chronicum migrans	Type IV

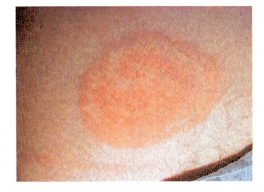

58 Reactive erythema in a child. These lesions (sometimes known as erythema annulare centrifugum) have erythematous borders and a dusky centre. They may occur anywhere on the skin, may be single or multiple, and usually enlarge slowly. Lesions may continue to appear over a period of several months. The mechanism in this form of reactive erythema is unclear, although Type I hypersensitivity is a likely cause in some cases. In infants the lesions may be associated with a maternal autoimmune disorder, such as systemic lupus erythematosus, and in older children they may follow a viral infection.

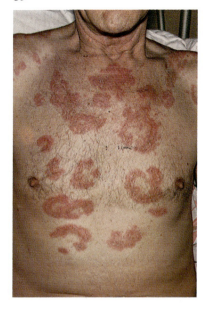

59 Erythema annulare centrifugum in an adult. On a single inspection this appearance might suggest a cutaneous reticulosis, such as B-cell lymphoma, but the behaviour of the lesions, with the disappearance of some over a period of time, is reassuring and suggests erythema annulare centrifugum. In case of doubt, however, skin biopsy would be essential to exclude malignant infiltration.

Atopic Eczema

Several immunological abnormalities have been identified in this condition. However, the overall pathogenesis is still unclear. A combination of both Type I and Type IV hypersensitivity reactions are thought to be involved (see also Chapters 7 and 10). Elevated serum and cutaneous IgE levels are the most consistent findings, indicating the involvement of a Type I mechanism in this common disorder. However, the level of IgE in the dermis does not always correlate with disease activity.

Lack of T-cell suppression may be responsible for the excessive IgE production. High levels of IgE sensitise mast cells to environmental antigens, e.g. from foods and house dust mite excreta. This results in excessive histamine release on subsequent contact with these allergens.

Histamine and other mediators from mast cells or basophils may be responsible for the acute inflammation seen in atopic eczema. The clinical appearances, however, are quite different from those seen in urticaria – presumably due to the multifactorial genesis of eczema.

Urticaria has a broadly similar clinical appearance and distribution in all age groups. In contrast, atopic eczema, even in the acute phase, has different characteristics in patients of different ages (**60–64**). The diagnosis and management of atopic eczema are fully discussed in Chapters 10 and 11.

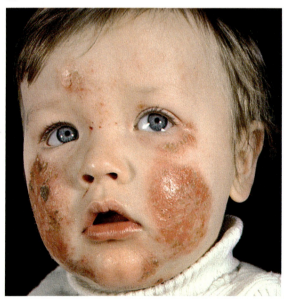

60 Atopic eczema in the infantile stage. Infants are rarely born with the condition, but typically develop the first signs of inflammation at about the age of 3 months – usually on the face, with typical involvement of the cheeks, sparing the perioral skin.

61 Atopic eczema in the acute phase typically affects the flexures – antecubital fossa, neck, wrists, and ankles. Development to this distribution usually occurs after the age of 2 years, although this infant developed eczema behind the knee at an earlier age.

62 Generalised infantile atopic eczema can be very widespread, as shown in this 3-year-old girl. In addition to disease in the flexures, there is a widespread eruption over the trunk and face, and some involvement of other areas of the limbs. In a small proportion of cases, allergy to food may be an aetiological factor in this phase, and the course of the disease may be influenced by life events, such as teething, stress, or respiratory infections.

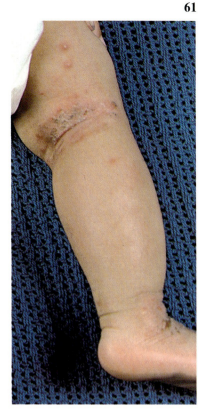

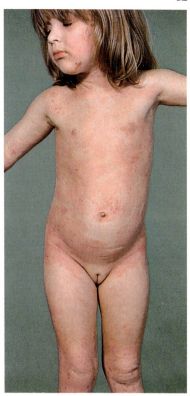

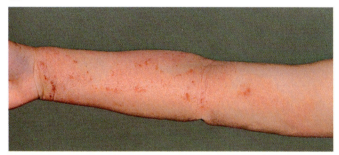

63 Atopic eczema is relatively rare after puberty, but when it persists it usually resumes its flexural distribution and may be complicated by secondary infection – as in this young girl who demonstrates marked excoriation and secondary impetigo.

64 Atopic eczema – facial involvement in a 59-year-old woman. This patient had a long history of eczema, but had relapsed just prior to this photograph being taken, with severe facial involvement and secondary bacterial infection. The mechanism of this type of acute exacerbation in adult eczema is unclear, but hormonal changes, stress, or intercurrent disease may play a role.

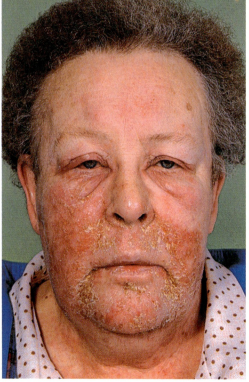

Allergic Rhinitis

Seasonal rhinitis is the commonest of all allergic diseases and is often associated with atopic eczema, urticaria, or conjunctivitis. Up to 20% of the population of western countries suffer from non-viral rhinitis, and about 50% of cases are allergic in origin. Allergic rhinitis may be *seasonal* or *perennial*.

The commonest cause of *seasonal* rhinitis is pollen allergy, but moulds are another cause of seasonal symptoms. The range of allergens in the air varies from time to time, and from place to place.

Perennial rhinitis is most commonly caused by allergy to the faeces of the house dust mite, though symptoms may show seasonal exacerbation, being worst during the winter when the mite population is greatest. Allergy to cats, dogs, horses, and other domestic animals may also cause perennial rhinitis, while occasional exposure may cause intermittent symptoms. Atopic eczema is a common association.

Patients with allergic rhinitis have positive skin prick tests and sometimes also an elevated serum IgE level. The reaction is IgE-mediated (Type I), though some patients can also be shown to have a late reaction which may involve Type IV mechanisms. Patients with similar symptoms who have negative skin prick tests and a normal serum IgE are said to have *non-specific rhinitis*. It is probable that some of these patients have a reaction to an unidentified allergen, and that others have an allergic reaction confined to the nose; but some may be hyper-reactive to irritants, such as airborne pollutants, rather than truly allergic.

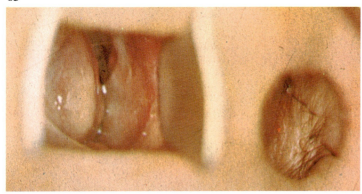

65 Acute rhinitis in seasonal allergy. The nasal mucous membrane is oedematous, so the inferior turbinate abuts against the septum, causing obstruction. A similar appearance is seen in perennial rhinitis and in the common cold, though the infected mucous membrane tends to be redder than that seen in allergy.

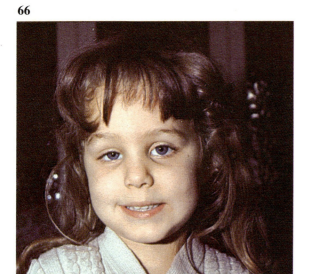
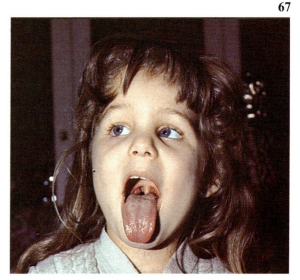

66–69 The characteristic facial appearance of a child with nasal allergy. This 5-year-old girl has infraorbital oedema and a characteristic gaping appearance of the mouth (**66**), through which she normally breathes as a result of nasal obstruction. Her large fleshy tonsils can be seen clearly (**67**).

Acute allergic rhinitis leads to oedematous changes in the nasal mucosa (**65**), and long-term or recurrent rhinitis may lead to characteristic facial appearances in children (**66–70**). These appearances should prompt inquiry into other possible manifestations of atopy, such as atopic eczema.

Seasonal and perennial rhinitis can be wholly or partially prevented by the use of regular nasal corticosteroid therapy. In seasonal rhinitis, the effect of this therapy is maximised if it is started before the onset of the provoking pollen season. Nasal sodium cromoglycate is occasionally helpful in nasal allergy, but for the full effect it must be administered six or more times per day, which limits its use. Oral antihistamine therapy is the mainstay of therapy for many patients. It has the advantage that it also improves accompanying conjunctival symptoms, and it may suppress urticaria or the itching from accompanying atopic eczema. Modern non-sedating antihistamines are free from the major side-effect (drowsiness) which previously limited the use of this group of drugs.

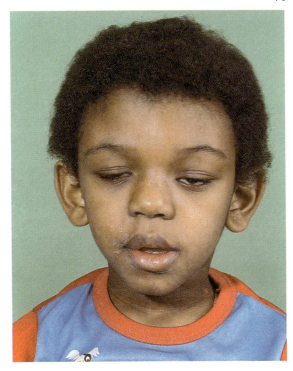

70 An atopic child. This 7-year-old boy's main problem was asthma, but he has characteristic atopic facies, with a lethargic expression, infraorbital and perioral oedema, a swollen and congested nose, and some facial eczema, especially around the mouth.

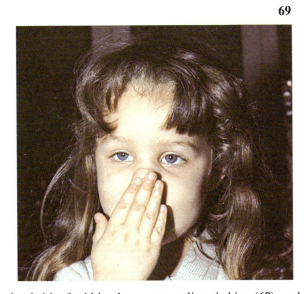

66–69 (*cont.*) She also has chronic rhinitis, as shown by her habit of rubbing her nose to relieve itching (**68**), and by the characteristic 'allergic salute', in which the fingers and palm of the hand are rubbed upwards over the tip of the nose (**69**).

Nasal Polyps

Nasal polyps are uncommon in both allergic and non-specific rhinitis, but they are characteristic of 'salicylate-associated rhinitis'. This syndrome usually consists of the triad of rhinitis with nasal polyps, sinusitis, and asthma, and all three conditions are exacerbated by aspirin and by other non-steroidal anti-inflammatory drugs (and by salicylate-rich foods). Some of these patients also have salicylate-provoked urticaria. The mechanism of this type of rhinitis is not fully understood. It is usually associated with eosinophilia, but the serum IgE level is normal, and skin tests are usually negative. A non-allergic mechanism is likely.

Nasal polyps may cause unremitting nasal obstruction and anosmia (**71, 72**). Surgical excision may be required, although polyps sometimes respond well to local or systemic corticosteroid treatment. This may need to be continued indefinitely to prevent recurrence.

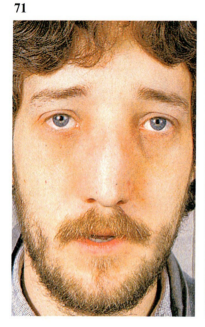
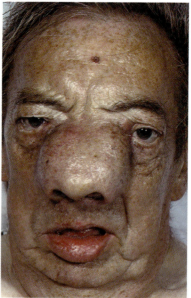

71 Nasal polyps, causing widening of the nose in a young man with asthma and urticaria – both provoked by salicylate and related non-steroidal anti-inflammatory drugs. Some patients with this condition also have salicylate-provoked urticaria.

72 Nasal polyposis. This patient provides an extreme example of long-standing nasal polyposis with gross widening of the nasal bones. These polyps had been slowly enlarging for many years, and there was no clear history of underlying salicylate sensitivity or other allergic disease. Treatment at this stage can only be surgical.

Immediate Allergic Reactions in the Eye

The eye is quite commonly involved in allergic skin disease, and it is also the site of some specific allergic reactions (*Table 15*).

Patients with urticaria and/or atopic eczema are particularly prone to IgE-mediated acute allergic conjunctivitis. Hay fever is the commonest cause, but similar symptoms may occur in response to other allergens. Patients who are allergic to cats or dogs, for example, frequently develop both acute allergic conjunctivitis and angioedema, and both symptoms may be exacerbated by rubbing allergen-contaminated fingers into itchy eyes.

In acute conjunctivitis due to hay fever or other causes the eyes appear normal between episodes. When signs are present they are usually mild, consisting of hyperaemia and slight swelling of the tarsal conjunctiva, with some chemosis of the vulvar conjunctiva (**73**). There are no long-term consequences.

Vernal catarrh is more serious and long-lasting. The condition is commonest in children between 5–15 years of age, and it usually remits in adult life. The typical patient has multiple positive skin prick tests to a broad range of allergens. The symptoms of vernal catarrh are much more severe than those of hay fever conjunctivitis. Itching is a major symptom, together with a copious discharge of lardaceous mucopurulent material. Photophobia can be extremely severe on waking in the morning, and children may often require periods of 30–45 minutes for adaptation to daylight. The signs of vernal catarrh are of large cobblestone papillae, and of muco-

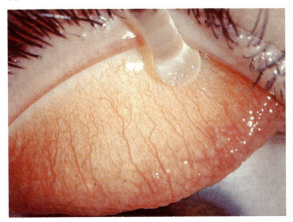

73 Hay fever conjunctivitis. The everted upper tarsal plate shows hyperaemia and oedema, but the vertical tarsal blood vessels are visible.

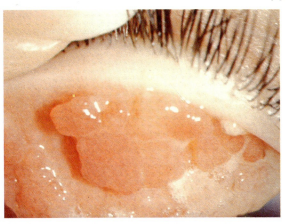

74 Active vernal catarrh, with large papillae on the everted upper tarsal plate. There is a copious discharge of mucopurulent material, associated with severe itching and photophobia.

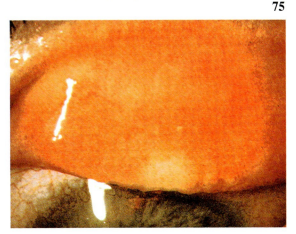

75 Atopic conjunctivitis. There are many fine papillae present in the everted upper tarsal plate. Hyperaemia and cellular infiltration disguise the anatomical structure of the normal tarsal blood vessels.

purulent discharge in the conjuctival sac (**74**). The active disease may be associated with the formation of micro-erosions in the upper half of the cornea, and this sign indicates a need for urgent treatment. Severe vernal catarrh can lead to chronic corneal ulceration, and can thus be a threat to sight. Referral to an ophthalmologist is required in these circumstances.

Atopic conjunctivitis (**75**) is often seen in atopic adults. The appearances in the tarsal plates are different to those seen in vernal catarrh in children, in that the papillae are fine and closely packed together, producing a hyperaemic 'felty' appearance of the upper tarsal plate, which disguises the usual anatomy of the vascular arcade. The symptoms are itching and a chronic discharge, and there may be a chronic keratitis. In some adult patients, severe herpetic keratitis can be a complicating problem.

Acute allergic eye disease may be prevented by regular use of sodium cromoglycate eye drops or ointment, and the symptoms may be treated with oral antihistamines. For regular use, non-sedating antihistamines have obvious advantages.

Severe Type I allergic eye disease may need treatment with corticosteroid eye drops, but these should only be prescribed under ophthalmological control.

Table 15. *Examples of hypersenstiivity reactions in the eye.*

Type I (immediate type)
Acute allergic conjunctivitis with conjunctival oedema in children
Hay fever conjunctivitis
Vernal keratoconjunctivitis
Atopic conjunctivitis in adults

Type II (cytotoxic type)
Pemphigus vulgaris
Cicatricial pemphigoid

Type III (immune-complex-mediated)
Scleritis (PAN, RA, SLE, etc.)
Erythema multiforme/Stevens–Johnson syndrome

Type IV (cell-mediated, delayed type)
Contact conjunctivitis
Phlyctenular keratoconjunctivitis
Corneal graft rejection

Mechanism uncertain
Contact lens-associated giant papillary conjunctivitis (GPC)
Peripheral corneal melting syndrome

Insect Sting Allergy

Reactions to venomous insect stings may result from immunological or non-immunological mechanisms. Insect venom itself may provoke a local reaction at the site of a sting, and this may closely resemble a local urticarial reaction, but the sting is usually painful and its nature is thus obvious.

Immediate, anaphylactic-type reactions involve an IgE-mediated mechanism. These may be dramatic, provoking severe angioedema (**53, 76–78**), asthma, anaphylaxis, and death. Prior sensitisation is required for such a response, so the first sting received by an individual never causes a reaction of this type, and life-threatening reactions are rare in childhood.

The response in a sensitised individual is complicated by the usual presence of IgG antibodies to the venom. These act as 'blocking antibodies' and – if present in adequate concentrations – may prevent an IgE-mediated response. Their level is not, however, consistent. Beekeepers who are stung regularly often report that the first sting of the season provokes the worst reaction; presumably, it also provokes a restoration of the IgG response and acts as a form of immunotherapy against the effects of subsequent stings.

Immunotherapy may be effective in suppressing the response of sensitised individuals to insect stings. This is a complex field, however, so specialist advice should be sought before such therapy is commenced.

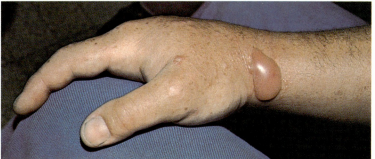

76 Bullous reaction to a wasp sting. Generalised swelling of the area surrounding the sting usually occurs and a bullous reaction is not uncommon. Note the generalised swelling of the affected hand in this patient. It is important to bear in mind the possibility of secondary infection, as wasps frequently feed on bacterially contaminated material.

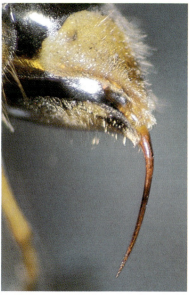

77 Wasp sting. This sting is a modified ovipositor (and therefore absent in males). It is composed of two lancets with fine subterminal barbs, a sheath, and a venom channel. Unlike the bee sting, the wasp sting can be withdrawn, and can thus inflict repeated wounds. The venom contains histamine, hyaluronidasse, serotonin, phospholipase A and B, various kinins, and other substances.

78 Severe angioedema in a 14-year-old girl following a bee sting. The patient required immediate treatment with adrenaline to overcome her anaphylactic response.

5 Skin Disorders Associated with Autoantibodies

Gell and Coombs' Type II humoral cytotoxic hypersensitivity reactions mainly involve IgG and IgM antibodies. They fix and activate complement when binding to foreign antigens, such as those on the surface of bacteria. When the antigen is coated with complement C_{3b} (opsonisation), it becomes easily phagocytosed by polymorphs and macrophages (see Chapter 2). Humoral cytotoxic reactions of this kind are typical of healthy defence against infectious agents, but they also mediate a range of autoimmune diseases.

The marker common to all autoimmune diseases is the presence of humoral autoantibodies. These probably reflect more basic defects of the immune system, such as the loss of T-lymphocyte suppressor activity. Immune complex damage is variable and is sometimes a secondary phenomenon. There is a failure to suppress the response to self antigens. Foreign antigens from microbes or drugs may share epitopes with self antigens. The unshared part of the foreign antigens may then bypass T-cell tolerance and in that way gain T-lymphocyte recognition, so stimulating a clone of B-lymphocytes, which react with both foreign and 'self' components.

Autoimmunity may affect single or multiple organs. Overlap between conditions occurs and the aetiology is usually unknown.

In the skin, diseases associated with cytotoxic autoantibodies fall into two groups – the primarily dermatological immunobullous disorders and the multisystem non-bullous disorders that cause dermatosis.

Immunobullous Disorders

The major immunobullous disorders are summarised in *Table 16*.

Table 16. *The major immunobullous disorders.*

	Site	History	Histology	Immunology	Other tests
Pemphigus	Mucous membranes and trunk	Insidious onset	Intra-epidermal blister	Direct IgG, C_3 Circulating IgG	
Pemphigoid	Upper arms and thighs	Blisters on eczematous base	Subepidermal blister	Fixed IgG and C_3 at dermoepidermal junction Circulating IgG	
Dermatitis herpetiformis	Scalp, scapula area, elbows, buttocks	Pruritus	Subepidermal blister	IgA in papillary dermis (granular)	Sub-total villous atrophy on jejunal biopsy
Linear IgA dermatosis	As in dermatitis herpetiformis or variable Perineum in children	Blistering lesions Usually non-pruritic	Subepidermal blister	IgA in papillary dermis (linear)	

Pemphigus

Pemphigus is a rare, potentially lethal, intra-epidermal blistering disease involving the skin and mucous membranes. It is caused by the attachment of circulating IgG antibodies to the intercellular substance of the epidermis.

The mildest form of the disease is pemphigus foliaceus (**79**). If localised, this variant is known as pemphigus erythematosus, and can be associated with systemic lupus erythematosus (SLE). There is no particular racial prevalence.

Generalised pemphigus vulgaris (and its variant pemphigus vegetans, which occurs in the flexures) is a more immediately dangerous condition. It is more common in Jews, and affects both sexes equally. Blisters may develop on mucous membranes (**12**) and skin (**80**).

Skin biopsy shows an intra-epidermal blister (**41**) and direct immunofluorescence confirms tissue-fixed intercellular IgG antibody in the epidermis (**42, 81**). The indirect test for circulating antibody requires substrate tissue, e.g. primate oesophagus or human vaginal mucosa. Following incubation with the patient's serum, fluorescein-labelled antibody to IgG and complement is applied. The serum can be diluted and the test can be quantified. The titre of circulating antibody correlates with the clinical activity of the disease.

Pemphigus vulgaris should be treated with high-dose systemic corticosteroids and antibiotics. In untreated pemphigus, secondary infection and fluid and electolyte imbalance can be fatal. Long-term treatment with corticosteroids or immunosuppressive drugs is often necessary.

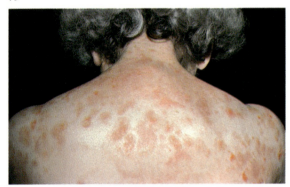

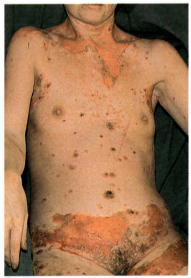

79 Pemphigus foliaceus is the mildest form of pemphigus and is often misdiagnosed due to the superficial nature of the lesions and the lack of clinical blistering. This elderly lady demonstrates the typical appearance, with evidence of superficial erosion and healing. Autoantibodies (usually IgG) can be found by immunofluorescence in the intercellular epidermal space. Curiously, however, the split is found at the subcorneal level. Pemphigus foliaceus is more likely than other forms of pemphigus to respond to corticosteroid therapy.

80 Pemphigus vulgaris. This potentially fatal condition can begin insidiously with mouth ulceration (**12**), which can persist for several weeks. Characteristically, as in this young woman, the condition progresses to a widespread eruption involving extensive raw areas and shallow erosions. Blisters are not always evident. Direct immunofluorescence studies show findings identical to those in pemphigus foliaceus, but light microscopy shows that the epidermal split in pemphigus vulgaris occurs at the suprabasal level.

81 Direct immunofluorescence in pemphigus. Note the intercellular epidermal deposition of IgG. C_3 and, occasionally, IgM may also be deposited. The sub-types of pemphigus are differentiated by light microscopy, and cannot be distinguished using direct immunofluorescence.

Pemphigoid

Pemphigoid, sometimes termed 'bullous pemphigoid' to distinguish it from cicatricial pemphigoid, usually affects patients over 60 years of age. Pruritus and urticated plaque formation may precede the bullous stage by several months (**82**). When blisters appear, they are usually generalised (**83**), but mucous membrane involvement is rare and transient. The blisters may bleed and they may become infected, requiring systemic antibiotic therapy.

The blisters are subepidermal – between the dermis and epidermis (**84**). As with pemphigus, tissue-fixed and circulating autoantibodies have been demonstrated, suggesting that the disease may have an autoimmune pathogenesis. Immunoglobulin and complement are found in a linear band at the dermoepidermal junction (**85**).

Treatment of pemphigoid usually requires long-term immunosuppression – most commonly with a combination of systemic corticosteroids and a steroid-sparing agent (such as azathioprine or methotrexate). Maintenance therapy is usually required for months or even years. Antihistamine therapy can be used to control itch, especially in the pre-bullous stage.

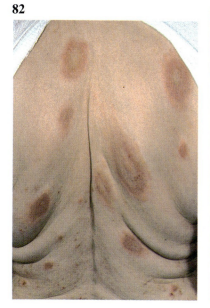
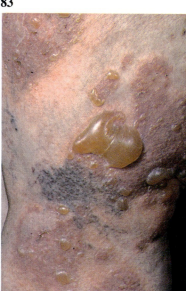
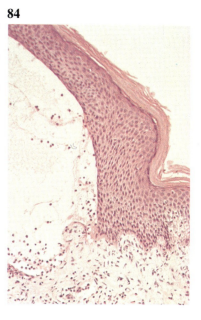

82 Pemphigoid typically presents in elderly patients, often with generalised pruritus, which may precede any blistering by several months. This patient has urticated plaques distributed over her trunk, which represent the pre-bullous stage of pemphigoid.

83 Pemphigoid. The same patient as in **82** later developed frank blisters containing fluid on an erythematous base. New blister formation can be clearly seen in the remaining urticated plaques. The split in pemphigoid is at the dermoepidermal junction.

84 Pemphigoid. Light microscopy shows clearly a subepidermal blister associated with an inflammatory reaction. Numerous eosinophils are often present.

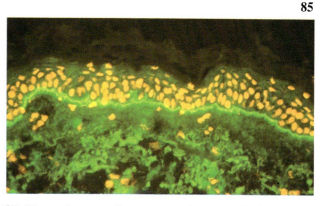

85 Direct immunofluorescence in pemphigoid reveals IgG deposition in the basement membrane, and the counterstain highlights the nuclei of the epidermal keratinocytes above. This test is best performed on perilesional skin biopsies, rather than on the blisters themselves. Granular deposition of C_3 is also often observed.

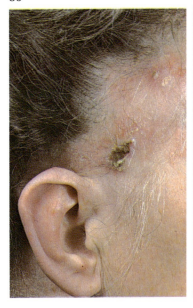
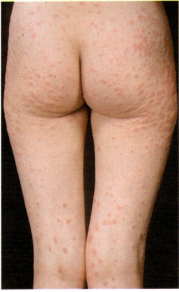

86 Cicatricial pemphigoid. This also affects elderly patients, and is also termed mucous membrane pemphigoid as it commonly affects the mucous membranes of the eyes, mouth, and sometimes the genitalia. In this patient, scalp lesions have caused scarring alopecia.

87 Herpes gestationis. This rare skin disorder presents with vesicles and bullae, and occurs during pregnancy and the puerperium. It can resemble bullous pemphigoid, but can sometimes be distinguished from it by immunofluorescence techniques. The condition tends to recur in subsequent pregnancies.

Cicatricial pemphigoid is also seen in elderly patients. It is a chronic blistering condition, affecting the mucous membranes and, sometimes, the skin (**86**). It often responds to dapsone therapy, but may require similar treatment to bullous pemphigoid.

Herpes gestationis

Herpes gestationis is a rare disease of pregnancy, which tends to recur in successive pregnancies. It usually presents with intense itching. Classically, it resembles bullous pemphigoid in its appearance (**87**), but at the other end of the clinical spectrum it merges into other eruptions of pregnancy, especially toxic urticated erythemas. The most common finding on direct immunoflourescence of perilesional skin is linear deposition of C_3 along the basement membrane zone. In 40% of patients, IgG is also found at the dermoepidermal junction. Complement-fixing IgG autoantibodies, the 'HG factor' have been isolated, but from fewer patients than for bullous pemphigoid. There are several reports of increased fetal death rate, and transient rashes and antibodies in the baby. In severe cases, this condition should be treated with systemic corticosteroids.

Dermatitis herpetiformis

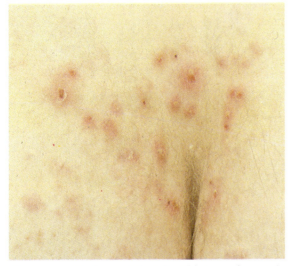

88 Dermatitis herpetiformis. This rare, intensely itchy symmetrical eruption typically occurs over the scalp, elbows, sacral area – as seen here – and buttocks (see **5**). Due to the intense itching, the condition often presents with excoriations rather than vesicles.

Dermatitis herpetiformis is an intensely pruritic blistering skin condition (**5, 88, 89**), associated with deposition of IgA in dermal papillae, and with gluten-sensitive enteropathy. Patients usually present in their third and fourth decades, and males are more commonly affected than females. The blisters are subepidermal and small compared with the larger lesions of bullous pemphigoid. No circulating antibody has yet been consistently found in dermatitis herpetiformis patients, but histology and direct

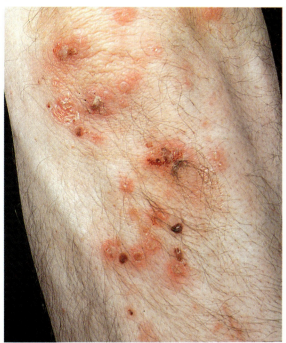

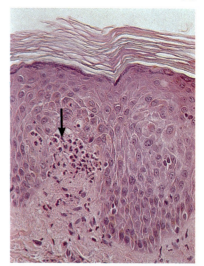

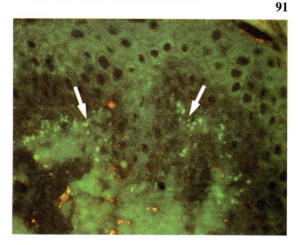

89 Dermatitis herpetiformis. In this patient, clustering of the erythematous vesicles is clearly seen over the extensor surface of the forearm. The split in dermatitis herpetifomis is subepidermal with characteristic immunofluorescence findings (**90, 91**).

90 Dermatitis herpetiformis. Light microscopy showing a typical papillary tip microabscess (arrowed). The split subsequently develops at the same subepidermal location.

91 Dermatitis herpetiformis. Immunofluorescence reveals IgA deposition in the papillary tips (arrowed) – at a site corresponding to the microabscesses on light microscopy (**90**). As in pemphigoid (**85**), the biopsy should be taken from perilesional skin. This abnormality on immunofluorescence may persist for several years, despite clinical resolution and normal light microscopic findings.

immunofluorescence of the skin are diagnostic (**90, 91**).

Most patients do not have overt symptoms or signs of malabsorption, but even so a jejunal biopsy should be performed to identify the sub-total villous atrophy, which is present in most cases. When this is present, it should be treated with a gluten-free diet. The lesions respond within 24–48 hours to dapsone and to a gluten-free diet over 2–3 years.

Linear IgA dermatosis

Linear IgA dermatosis may present in exactly the same way as dermatitis herpetiformis, but it may also resemble bullous pemphigoid or other blistering conditions. It occurs at all ages and, in childhood, has been termed benign chronic bullous disease of childhood (**92–94**). There is no association between linear IgA dermatosis and gluten enteropathy. Direct immunofluorescence on skin biopsy shows a linear rather than a granular pattern of IgA deposition, but this is at the same subepidermal location as the granular deposits in dermatitis herpetiformis. Dapsone or sulphapyridine may suppress the condition, but systemic corticosteroid therapy may be needed occasionally.

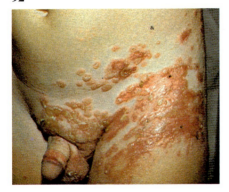

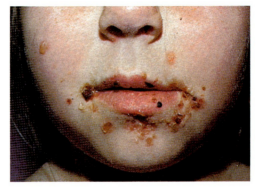

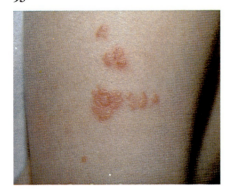

92 Linear IgA dermatosis. This rare inflammatory blistering disorder typically occurs in the perineum and surrounding areas in children. Pruritus is usually mild (unlike dermatitis herpetiformis) and lesions can assume an annular configuration, with blisters forming the outer border of the ring.

93 Linear IgA dermatosis. This patient has ring-like blisters on the leg typical of linear IgA dermatosis. The light microscopic findings can be indistinguishable from those in pemphigoid, but immunofluorescence is diagnostic, showing a linear distribution of IgA, rather than the granular appearance seen in dermatitis herpetiformis.

94 Linear IgA dermatosis. Inflammatory blisters around the mouth may be misdiagnosed as bullous impetigo. In linear IgA dermatosis they rarely occur in isolation; this emphasises the importance of examining the whole patient.

Non-bullous Dermatoses

Multisystem autoimmune disorders

A number of multisystem disorders are caused by or associated with circulating autoantibodies. Some are associated with HLA DR3 (*Table 17*), possibly because a gene linked to this tissue-type may result in inappropriate immune responsiveness. Some of these disorders commonly present with dermatological abnormalities. Most have some dermatological features.

Some autoimmune disorders involve more than one immune mechanism. Often, tissue damage follows binding of cytotoxic antibodies (Type II reaction) and from immune complex deposition (Type III). Rheumatoid arthritis is a good example of this dual pathophysiology. Along with other predominantly immune complex disorders, it is included in Chapter 6. In this chapter we examine conditions which primarily result from cytotoxic (Type II) reactions.

Table 17. *Diseases in which HLA-DR3 may be associated with autoimmune reactions.*

• Systemic lupus erythematosus
• Sjögren's syndrome
• Addison's disease
• Chronic hepatitis
• Myasthenia gravis
• Graves' disease

Lupus erythematosus

Lupus erythematosus (LE), as found in the skin, is now classified into three subtypes on the basis of antinuclear antibodies, photosensitivity, and systemic disease (*Table 18*).

Table 18. *Subtypes of lupus erythematosus.*

	Antinuclear Antibody	Sun Sensitivity	Systemic Involvement
Discoid	+	+	–
Subacute LE	+	++++	+
SLE	+++	+++	++

Discoid LE

Discoid lupus should not be confused with subacute LE or with systemic LE (SLE), in which general health is affected and major laboratory abnormalities are found. The skin is always affected in discoid lupus, but it is not always affected in the systemic form. Progression from discoid lupus to SLE is rare.

The skin lesions in discoid LE are characteristically slowly-enlarging plaques, which occur mainly in light-exposed areas (**95–97**) and, if untreated, result in permanent scarring.

Photosensitivity contributes to the progression of discoid LE, and its treatment must include strict sun avoidance and the use of sunscreens. Topical corticosteroids and, in resistant cases, a short course of antimalarial therapy – e.g. hydroxychloroquine – may be used for a short time, during the summer months only, to avoid eye complications.

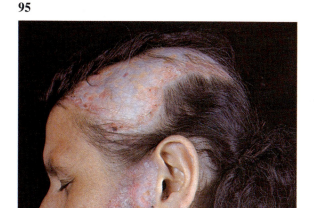

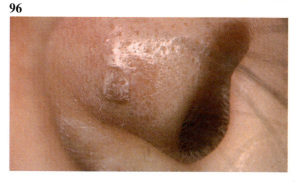

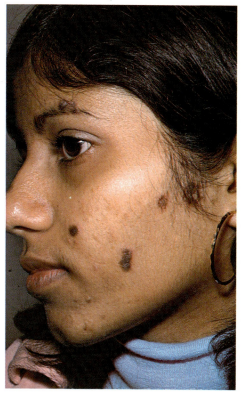

95 Discoid lupus erythematosus. This patient has slowly enlarging pink scaly plaques on the scalp that extend onto the face. The disease tends to occur in light-exposed areas. If left untreated, the condition can lead to severe permanent scarring, as in this unfortunate Asian lady.

96 Discoid lupus erythematosus. In this disorder the pilosebaceous follicles are characteristically plugged with keratin. This is usually evident in the ear, as seen here.

97 Discoid lupus erythematosus. This patient demonstrates a much earlier stage in the disease and, due to her skin colour, the plaques tend to be rather hyperpigmented. At this stage, the diagnosis requires confirmation by biopsy.

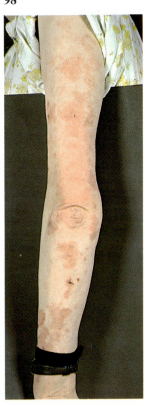

Subacute LE

This subtype of LE usually presents with symmetrical, sharply marginate, scaly, sometimes annular or even urticated plaques, mainly with a photosensitive distribution (**98**). It can be difficult to distinguish from disseminated discoid LE, but there is little or no scarring and systemic disease is frequent in subacute LE. Deposition of immunoglobulin in the skin, as demonstrated by immunofluorescence, is less common in subacute LE than in discoid LE or in SLE. Serum autoantibodies are present less often in subacute LE than in SLE, but many patients have antibodies to extractable nuclear antigens, particularly anti Ro/SSA. As in SLE, neonatal LE can occur in babies born to mothers with subacute LE. The skin lesions are temporary, but permanent heart block is a serious complication of subacute LE. Treatment with sunscreens, systemic corticosteroids, and/or antimalarials or dapsone is often required.

98 Subacute lupus erythematosus. This patient has widespread urticarial-like erythematous plaques, occurring in light-exposed areas. Investigations revealed a positive antinuclear antibody and anti-Ro antibody. She responded well to topical sunscreens and dapsone.

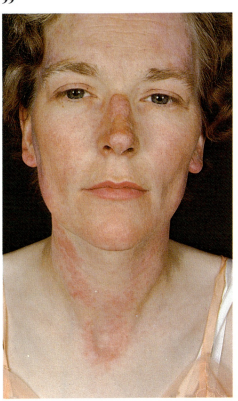

Systemic LE

Cutaneous signs of SLE include a butterfly rash on the face (**99**), diffuse alopecia which is non-scarring, mucosal ulceration, nail-fold telangiectasia and erythema (**13**), Raynaud's phenomenon (**100**), and discrete palpable purpuric lesions signifying vasculitis. Patients often present with systemic symptoms, such as malaise, fever, and arthralgia. The aetiology is usually unknown, but the disease may be drug-induced, especially in slow acetylators.

Multisystem involvement is characteristic of SLE, and the most common cause of death in patients with the condition is renal failure. The prevalence of complications in SLE is summarised in *Table 19*. Diagnostic investigations include antinuclear antibodies (**43**) and the identification of LE cells (**45**).

99 Systemic lupus erythematosus (SLE). This middle-aged lady shows a typical 'butterfly' rash over the cheeks and bridge of the nose. She also shows changes on the forehead and around the neck, in light-exposed areas. These changes result from the photosensitivity which is commonly seen in this condition. Note the lack of scarring.

100 Systemic lupus erythematosus. This 32-year-old lady demonstrates typical Raynaud's phenomenon, which commonly occurs in non-bullous autoimmune disorders. Note the bluish discoloration of the fingers, which were tender and cold to the touch. Severe Raynaud's phenomenon can result in gangrene.

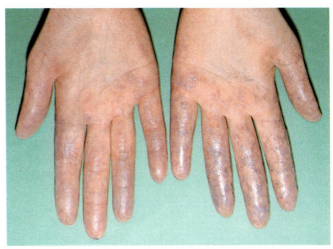

Treatment involves systemic corticosteroids and/or immunosuppressive drugs, and the prognosis has improved greatly in recent years. This makes the management of the skin manifestations of the disease particularly important. In addition to systemic therapy, it is essential that the patient does not become over-exposed to sunlight. Regular use of sunscreens is essential.

Table 19. *The prevalence of complications in patients with SLE at the time of diagnosis.*

	American Rheumatism Association prevalence (%)	UK prevalence (%)
Facial erythema	64	62
Discoid lupus	17	30
Raynaud's phenomenon	20	19
Alopecia	43	62
Photosensitivity	37	16
Oral/nasopharyngeal ulceration	15	22
Arthritis without deformity	90	86
LE cells	92	73
Chronic false positive serological tests for syphilis	12	8
Proteinuria (3.5 g/24 h)	20	24
Cellular casts in urine	48	16
Pleuritis and/or pericarditis	60/19	30/19
Psychosis and/or convulsions	19	19
Haematological abnormalities, one or more of:		
haemolytic anaemia	16	14
leucopenia	40	46
thrombocytopenia	11	14

* A positive score of four or more of the complications shown here confirms the diagnosis of SLE.

Scleroderma

Scleroderma is a condition characterised by fibrosis and contraction of connective tissue in the skin and in internal organs. A local form – morphoea – affects the skin alone. A generalised form – systemic sclerosis – affects many parts of the body. Where systemic sclerosis is accompanied by calcinosis and other features, it is often known as the CREST syndrome (Calcinosis, Raynaud's phenomenon, (o)Esophageal involvement, Sclerodactyly, and Telangiectasia).

Morphoea

This a localised form of scleroderma in the skin (**101, 102**). Rarely, the growth of underlying structures may be affected or severe atrophy and scarring may occur, as when the skin of the forehead and scalp is affected, giving the appearance of the scar of a sabre cut – '*en coup de sabre*' (**103**). Spontaneous resolution may occur but scarring may remain. No treatment is helpful.

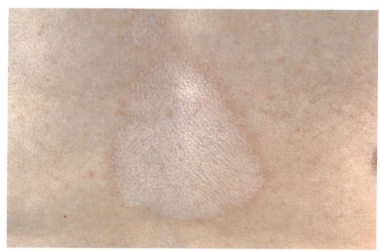

101 Localised morphoea. This young man presented with a pruritic plaque on the back. Note the hypopigmentation surrounded by an erythematous hue, an appearance that is very typical in the early stage of the disorder. There is no systemic involvement.

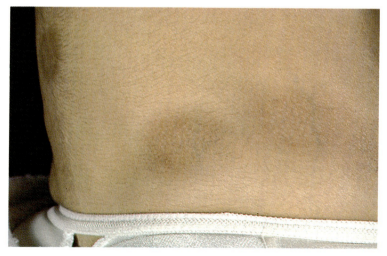

102 Localised morphoea. In this young Asian lady, several hyperpigmented plaques developed insidiously over the trunk. Note the superficial atrophic changes, which are typical of the later stages of the disease. The changes in pigmentation are often dependent on the patient's skin type, and do not reflect disease activity.

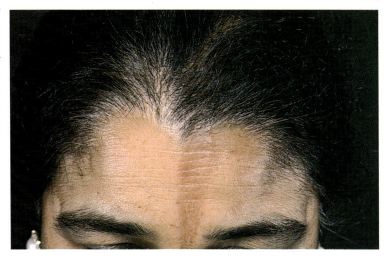

103 *En coup de sabre.* This form of localised morphoea can involve subcutaneous tissues and even bone. It is a variant of linear morphoea and, if the scalp is involved, can be associated with scarring and subsequent hair loss. Despite the severe local involvement, systemic sclerosis is not seen in this condition.

Systemic sclerosis

In contrast to morphoea, this is a serious multisystem disease. Patients are usually female. They present with Raynaud's phenomenon and/or dysphagia, or with features of the CREST syndrome – see above and (**104–106**). The heart, lungs, kidney, and gastrointestinal tract may be involved. Occasionally, a culminating variety leads to rapid death. Positive investigations include high titres of antinuclear factor, and abnormal oesophageal motility. Lung, liver, and renal functions may all be affected. Treatment is disappointing. Potassium aminobenzoate, penicillamine, and systemic corticosteroids have been used in therapy with varying results. Physiotherapy and thermoregulation are often helpful in symptomatic relief, as are H_2-receptor antagonists for symptoms of oesophageal reflux.

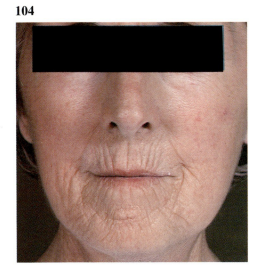

104 Systemic sclerosis. This middle-aged lady has characteristic features of scleroderma involving the perioral skin, which is tight, shiny, and puckered, with several telangiectasia around the mouth and on the cheeks. She was unable to open her mouth widely, and she had accompanying sclerodactyly, Raynaud's phenomenon (see **100**), rigidity of the oesophagus, and calcinosis of the fingers (see **105**) – the CREST syndrome.

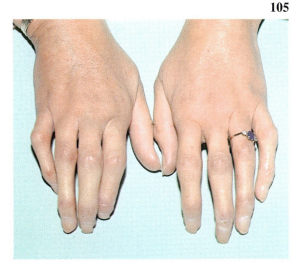

105 Systemic sclerosis with calcinosis of the fingers, showing palpable nodules and ulceration of the fingertips on clinical examination.

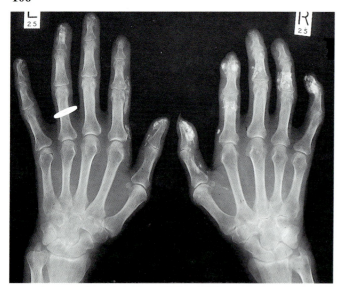

106 An X-ray of the systemic sclerosis shown in **105**, illustrating the extensive subcutaneous soft tissue calcification in both hands.

Dermatomyositis

This is a rare condition which may be associated with an underlying malignancy – usually an adenocarcinoma. Characteristic skin changes include a heliotrope (purplish) erythema and oedema of the face (**105**), violaceous plaques on extensor surfaces of limb joints, and nail-fold changes (**13, 108**). Proximal muscle weakness and pain occur due to a polymyositis. Electromyography and muscle biopsy may aid diagnosis. Serum creatine phosphokinase is usually elevated. Hypergammaglobulinaemia, rheumatoid factor, antinuclear factor, and false positive tests for syphilis can occasionally be found.

Dermatomyositis seems to result from immune-mediated vessel injury, in which complement is bound and activated in arterioles and capillaries – mainly in muscle tissue.

Underlying malignancy is common. If no obvious tumour is found, lungs, prostate, breasts, and pelvic organs should be investigated. Most underlying tumours are not easily treatable, but the skin and muscle symptoms may respond to systemic corticosteroid or other immunosuppressive treatment.

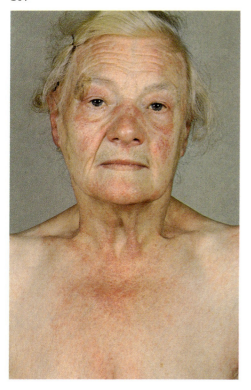

107 Dermatomyositis. This elderly lady has characteristic erythema and oedema of the face, with purple discoloration of the eyelids – termed a 'heliotrope' appearance. Note that the eruption extends onto the V of the neck, and could easily be confused with a light-sensitive eruption. She also complained of proximal muscle weakness. Investigation revealed that she had an underlying carcinoma of the bronchus.

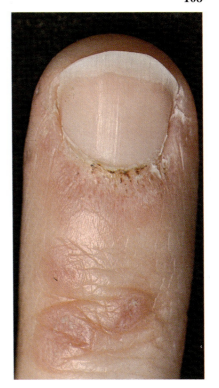

108 Dermatomyositis. Nail-fold erythema and telangiectasia with ragged cuticles are useful physical signs of non-bullous non-organ-specific autoimmune disorders, and are commonly seen in dermatomyositis and in SLE. Violaceous plaques and papules may also occur on the knuckles, knees, and elbows in dermatomyositis.

Relapsing polychondritis

This is an uncommon condition characterised by recurrent episodes of inflammation of the cartilage and related tissues (**109**). The ears, eyes, joints, nose, larynx, trachea, and cardiovascular system can be involved. Respiratory or cardiovascular involvement can be fatal and a cytotoxic autoimmune pathogenesis is suspected. Autoantibodies to Type II collagen can be identified, and IgG and C_3 have been shown by immunofluorescence to be present in the affected cartilage. Immuosuppressive drugs may be helpful, and dapsone can sometimes help in mild cases.

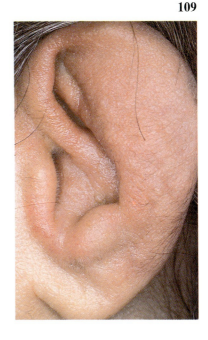

109 Relapsing polychondritis. This 45-year-old woman presented with a 3-week history of red eyes and pain in her anterior chest wall and ears. Note the erythema and swelling of the ear. The ear lobe is spared, as the underlying condition affects cartilage, which is present only in the pinna. The eyes are inflamed due to scleritis, because of the structural chemical similarities between the globe of the eye and cartilage. The anterior chest wall tenderness is the result of costal cartilage involvement. Other physical signs can include hoarseness of the voice due to laryngeal cartilage involvement, and tenderness and collapse of the nose.

Organ-Specific Autoimmune Disorders with Skin Manifestations

A number of organ-specific autoimmune disorders may present with skin manifestations. Some are reviewed here. It is important to remember that these disorders may coexist with each other or with multisystem disorders.

Hashimoto's disease (autoimmune thyroiditis)

This condition affects mainly middle-aged women and is associated with various autoantibodies. It may present early with transient thyrotoxicosis, or later with hypothyroidism.

Although not primarily a skin disorder, Hashimoto's disease may present with skin manifestations (**110**). Treatment with thyroxine usually results in gradual reversal of the skin changes.

110

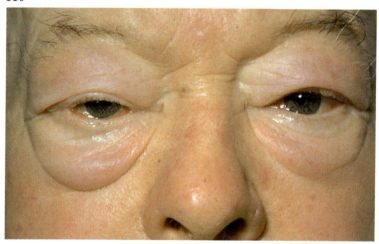

110 Hashimoto's disease usually presents with the features of hypothyroidism, but may be associated with oedematous changes in the face, especially periorbitally. It is important not to confuse these changes with dermatomyositis or even angioedema. The periorbital changes are constant rather than transient, and a firm nodular goitre is usually palpable in the neck.

111

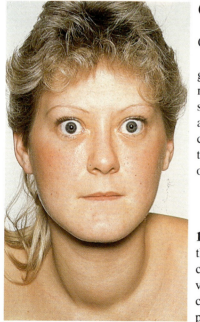

Graves' disease

Graves' disease is also not primarily a skin disorder.

Patients with Graves' disease are thyrotoxic. They develop a diffuse goitre, exophthalmos, and eyelid lag (**111**), and occasionally pre-tibial myxoedema (**112**). Investigation reveals a TSH-like IgG. Pituitary TSH is suppressed. The presence of 'long-acting thyroid stimulator' (LATS), acting on the whole gland and other tissues, helps to explain the various clinical features, which are not purely a consequence of elevated levels of thyroxine or tri-iodothyronine. Treatment involves suppressing thyroid overactivity with drugs, radioactive iodine, or surgery.

111 Graves' disease usually affects women between the ages of 20 and 40 years. This patient presented classically with a diffuse goitre, over which a vascular bruit could be heard, associated with the classic 'thyroid stare', which results from exophthalmos and lid retraction.

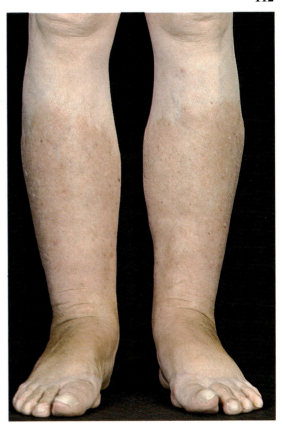

112 Pre-tibial myxoedema in a middle-aged lady with Graves' disease. The brawny, non-pitting swelling of the lower legs is typical of the dermatological changes in this condition. The dermatological changes do not always respond to reversal of the hyperthyroidism, but topical or intra-lesional corticosteroids may be helpful.

Addison's disease

Atrophy of the adrenal gland in the presence of autoantibodies is now the most common cause of deficient corticosteroid production. Patients present with weakness, anorexia, and gastrointestinal upset. Occasionally, they may be hypotensive, hypoglycaemic, and hypothermic, with vitiligo and alopecia. If the disease is not treated, coma and death may result.

The characteristic skin manifestation is hyperpigmentation, especially in skin creases and scars (**113**). Similar changes may occur in mucous membranes (**114**). These changes result from excessive production of ACTH by the pituitary – not directly from an immune process.

Treatment is based on glucocorticoid and mineralocorticoid replacement.

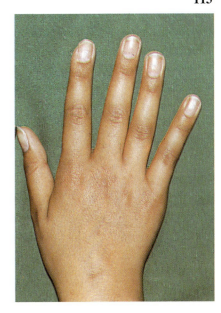

113 Addison's disease. This Caucasian patient noticed darkening of her skin and, on examination, was found to have hyperpigmentation, especially of her skin creases and in scars. Note the changes over the extensor surfaces of the interphalangeal joints. Similar changes can be seen in the palmar creases and in the buccal membrane (see **114**).

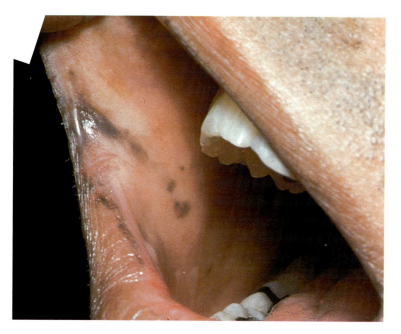

114 Addison's disease affects the buccal mucous membrane. There is a generalised hyperpigmentation of the membrane, with focal areas of deep pigmentation, which also occur on the lips. This increase in pigmentation is associated with increased ACTH levels; it does not result directly from an immunological process.

Pernicious anaemia

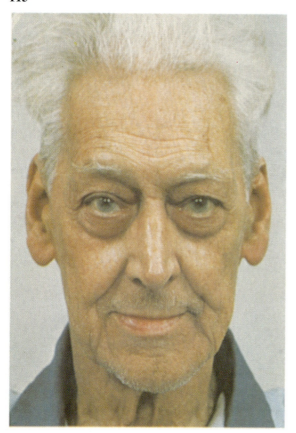

This is primarily a disease of the gastric mucosa in elderly patients. The stomach fails to produce hydrochloric acid, pepsin, and intrinsic factor. Gastric cytoplasmic antibodies are present in 80% of patients. Vitamin B_{12} is not absorbed in the absence of gastric intrinsic factor. As a result, patients may develop a macrocytic anaemia, with multilobular granulocytes and thrombocytopenia. Skin manifestations include pallor and a sallow pigmentation associated with the anaemia, and prematurely or completely grey hair (**115**). Patients characteristically have blue eyes, though the disease may occur in other groups (e.g. in young black women in the USA). Rarely, subacute degeneration of the cord may occur. Serum B_{12} levels and the Schilling test confirm the diagnosis. Treatment involves B_{12} replacement.

115 Pernicious anaemia. This patient showed a classic combination of anaemic pallor, lemon–yellow pigmentation, blue eyes, and grey hair. His tongue was also smooth and sore. Investigations revealed a megaloblastic anaemia, with a low serum B_{12} level. Gastric cytoplasmic antibodies were present in the serum.

6 Skin Disorders Associated with Immune Complexes

Vasculitis

The term vasculitis should be reserved for conditions which show inflammation within the vessel wall, with endothelial cell swelling, necrosis, and/or fibrinoid change. The clinical manifestation in the skin depends upon the size of the blood vessel affected and the type of cellular infiltrate. Many such disorders are immune-complex mediated and arise as a consequence of Type III hypersensitivity. Antigen may combine with antibodies near vital tissues, which are then damaged by the ensuing inflammatory responses. When an antigen is injected intradermally, for example, it combines with the appropriate antibodies on the walls of blood vessels. The complement pathway is then activated, generating C_{5a} which attracts polymorphonuclear leucocytes (the Arthus reaction). Degranulation of polymorphs liberates lysosomal enzymes which damage the vessel walls.

Antigen–antibody complexes may also be formed in the circulation and become deposited in the smaller vessels in the skin. Complement is then activated and inflammatory cells injure the vessels, as in the Arthus reaction. This vessel damage causes oedema and the extravasation of red blood cells results in the palpable purpura which characterises vasculitis clinically.

Leucocytoclastic vasculitis

Leucocytoclastic vasculitis is a relatively common disorder and is due to the deposition of immune complexes in the postcapillary venules. It is often referred to by other terms, such as allergic or hypersensitivity vasculitis or anaphylactoid purpura.

Crops of lesions arise in dependent areas – the legs and sometimes the forearms (**6, 116, 117**). Some may necrose and have livid, black, or ulcerated centres. Henoch–Schönlein purpura is a small vessel vasculitis, usually affecting children, associated with palpable purpura (**118**), arthritis, abdominal pain, and glomerulonephritis, and often preceded by an upper respiratory tract infection. Again, a necrotising vasculitis may ensue (**119**).

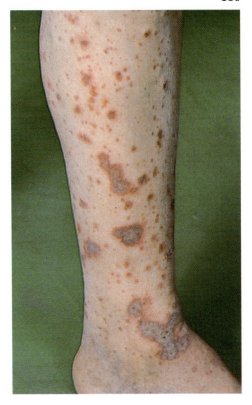

116 Leucocytoclastic vasculitis. This 57-year-old lady developed widespread palpable purpura on both legs. Although initially the lesions were scattered and discrete, by the time this photograph was taken, some had begun to coalesce and become necrotic in the centre. Urine tests revealed haematuria, which suggested renal involvement in the vasculitic process. Leucocytoclastic vasculitis can result from many causes. In this case, the underlying diagnosis was rheumatoid arthritis, and corticosteroid treatment was required to bring the vasculitis under control.

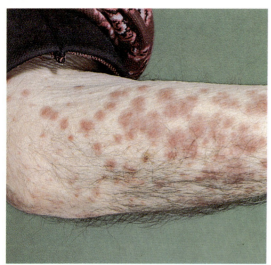

117 Leucocytoclastic vasculitis. In this elderly man the clinical appearance of the palpable purpura is different to that in **116**, as the individual lesions are larger and, in places, they resemble the annular lesions of erythema multiforme (see **132** and **133**). Skin biopsy confirmed that the underlying diagnosis was leucocytoclastic vasculitis. Despite an extensive vasculitic screen, no underlying cause was identified in this patient. The lesions were controlled with dapsone.

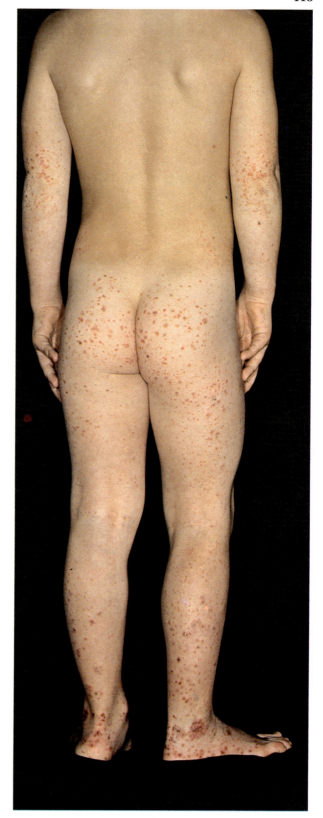

118 Henoch–Schönlein purpura is a small-vessel vasculitis which mainly affects children. The palpable purpuric lesions are most commonly found on the lower extremities and buttocks, but they may also appear on the arms, face, and ears. The trunk is usually spared. This patient had microscopic haematuria, and renal biopsy showed mesangial proliferative glomerulonephritis with some crescent formation. Acute nephritic symptoms are common in Henoch–Schönlein purpura, but the prognosis is good; only a small proportion of patients develop progressive renal failure.

119 Necrotising vasculitis may develop from Henoch–Schönlein or other forms of vasculitic purpura. In this child, the vasculitic lesions have coalesced in places over the buttocks, and numerous macules and papules with necrotic centres can be seen. Similar appearances may occur in septicaemic patients with a range of infections, including meningococcal and gonococcal infections, and infective endocarditis. Appropriate blood cultures and other investigations should always be performed where such an infection is a possibility.

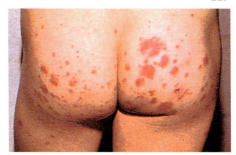

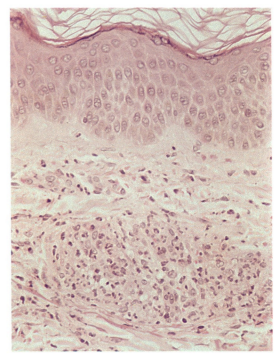

120 Skin biopsy in leucocytoclastic vasculitis (the same patient as shown in **116**). Note the intense perivascular mixed inflammatory infiltrate, consisting of numerous polymorphonuclear leucocytes. The small blood vessels are difficult to identify. There is extensive 'nuclear dust', which represents fragments of disintegrating neutrophils. The purpura seen clinically is due to the extravasation of red cells. Immunofluorescence in early lesions reveals immune-complex deposition within the blood vessel walls.

In all cases it is important to establish whether the vasculitis is simply cutaneous or systemic. Systemic vasculitis may affect the kidney, gastrointestinal tract, joints, lungs, and nervous system. The differential diagnosis should include other causes of purpura, such as coagulation abnormalities and sepsis. Occasionally, vasculitis may appear urticarial if purpura is not marked. Skin biopsy of early lesions (12 hours) with immunofluorescence may be diagnostic (**120**). IgA deposition in blood vessels is characteristic of patients with Henoch–Schönlein purpura.

Leucocytoclastic vasculitis may be caused by many different disorders (*Table 20*). Investigation of an unexplained vasculitis may reveal a treatable cause, and a routine sequence of investigations ('a vasculitis screen') should be performed whenever the underlying diagnosis is obscure (*Table 21*).

Table 20. *Aetiological factors in leucocytoclastic vasculitis.*

Infections	*Systemic disease*
Streptococcal infection	Non-organ-specific auto-
Hepatitis B	immune disorders, e.g. SLE,
Influenza	rheumatoid arthritis
Mononucleosis	Chronic active hepatitis
Cytomegalovirus	and biliary cirrhosis
Tuberculosis	Ulcerative colitis
Candidiasis	
Histoplasmosis	*Malignant disease*
	Hodgkin's disease
Drugs and chemicals	Multiple myeloma
Penicillin	Histiocytic lymphoma
Sulphonamide	Chronic lymphocytic
Aspirin	leukaemia
Quinidine	Hairy cell leukaemia
Allopurinol	Rare solid tumours
Iodides	
Insecticides and herbicides	
Hyposensitisation antigens	

Table 21. *Vasculitis screen.*

History	Investigation
Joint pain	Blood count
Abdominal pain	ESR
Blood in stool	Biochemical profile
Dyspnoea	Urinalysis for proteinuria and haematuria
Drug ingestion	Autoantibodies
Hyposensitisation therapy	Hepatitis antigen and antibody
Insecticide exposure	Chest X-ray
Hepatitis	
Recent upper respiratory tract infection	

N.B. Other tests may be indicated from histology, examination, or abnormal results of the investigations above.

Management of leucocytoclastic vasculitis

The management of vasculitis depends on the extent and severity of the lesions, and particularly on whether the function of involved organs is compromised. Immunosuppression with prednisolone and/or cyclophosphamide may be required. Sometimes either colchicine or dapsone can be helpful. Elimination of the suspected antigen and/or treatment of the underlying disease is always indicated.

Livedo vasculitis

Livedo vasculitis is a small vessel vasculitis and is also termed segmental hyalinising vasculitis. The pathological process involved is similar to that seen in leucocytoclastic vasculitis, but the process tends to occur at a deeper level in livedo vasculitis – hence the difference in clinical appearance. Lesions typically occur on the lower legs and ankles as stellate-shaped ulcers on an erythematous base and surrounded peripherally by a livedo reticularis (marble-like) pattern (**121**). Systemic lupus erythematosus (SLE) and other autoimmune disorders must be ruled out.

121

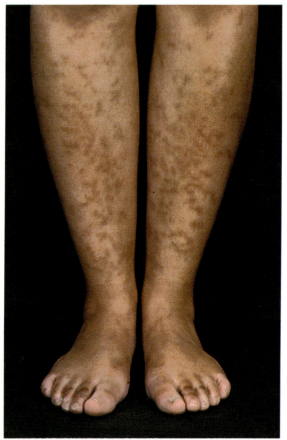

121 Livedo vasculitis. This 23-year-old Asian lady presented with a slowly developing mottled pigmentation of her legs. Note the characteristic livedo or 'reticular' appearance, resulting from the deeper level of involvement in livedo vasculitis. This patient's eruption proved to be a presenting feature of systemic lupus erythematosus (see Chapter 5).

Schamberg's disease

Schamberg's disease must be distinguished from leucocytoclastic vasculitis. Its distribution is similar, as it appears most commonly on the lower extremities; and at first sight it may look similar clinically. Multiple petechiae occur in a progressive manner, and they are followed by patches of brownish pigmentation due to haemosiderin deposition in the skin (**122**). The most characteristic feature is the presence of orange–brown, pinhead-sized 'cayenne pepper' spots (**123**).

The lesions may persist for months or years, but Schamberg's disease is benign – it is not accompanied by other systemic or local disease. Camouflage treatment may be required if the lesions are cosmetically disfiguring.

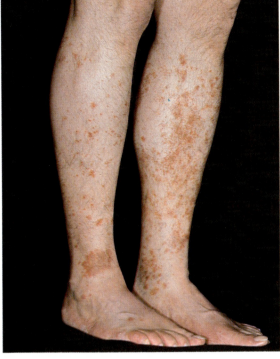

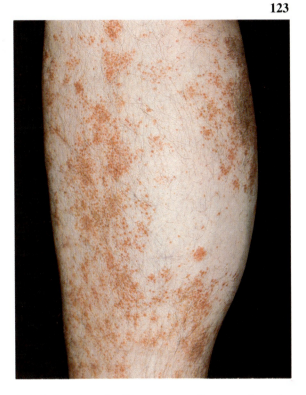

122 Schamberg's disease. In this condition, asymptomatic irregular orange–brown patches of varying shapes and sizes occur – most commonly on the lower limbs. The lesions are benign, and they are not accompanied by systemic disease; nor are there any venous or other disorders in the legs.

123 Schamberg's disease. In a close-up view, the most characteristic feature of the disease is seen – the orange–brown, pinhead-sized 'cayenne pepper' spots.

Urticarial vasculitis

Urticarial vasculitis is a rare form of vasculitis which may clinically resemble urticaria (see Chapter 4), but the individual lesions tend to be smaller than in urticaria, last longer than 24 hours, and may leave bruising in their wake (**124**). The relatively fixed urticarial lesions are accompanied by systemic symptoms, including arthralgias and abdominal pain. Lack of resolution can be determined by marking the outline of lesions with a pen and observing their progress. Skin biopsy reveals a sparse neutrophilic perivascular infiltrate in early lesions, with mild features of leucocytoclastic vasculitis. Direct immunofluorescence confirms that urticarial vasculitis is an immune-complex disease, usually showing deposition of granular immunoglobulins and complement within the superficial vessel walls. Total serum complement levels may be low; but – in contrast to leucocytoclastic vasculitis – significant renal disease is unusual. The condition tends to be chronic and recurrent, but may remit within several weeks. Indomethacin may be helpful in treatment, with or without systemic corticosteroids. Antihistamines are not usually beneficial.

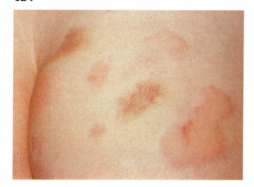

124 Urticarial vasculitis. In this patient, urticarial weals, which developed acutely, did not resolve for several days. Instead, they left a rather bruised, purpuric appearance. This is completely atypical of urticaria, but typical of urticarial vasculitis. The patient was generally unwell, with arthralgia and abdominal pain. The skin lesions are typical of Type III vasculitic lesions. These present with weals, which may be identical initially with the weals of urticaria, although individual lesions tend to be smaller in urticarial vasculitis. This patient required treatment with systemic corticosteroids. No underlying cause was identified.

Pyoderma gangrenosum

Pyoderma gangrenosum is a poorly understood ulcerating skin condition in which vasculitis can be identified in the perilesional skin, but it is still debatable whether the vasculitis is primary or secondary in these lesions. It most commonly occurs in patients with underlying chronic inflammatory or malignant disease, e.g. inflammatory bowel disease, rheumatoid arthritis, IgA monoclonal gammopathy, and reticulosis. The lesions may be preceded by minor trauma, which are often on the legs but can occur anywhere. They start as pustules or vesicles and quickly develop into indurated necrotic ulcers with a purulent base. A characteristic violaceous undermined edge and surrounding erythema occur (**125, 126**). Healing can take years and leaves a 'cribiform' pattern of scarring. Skin biopsy usually shows no specific changes: there is abscess formation with evidence of vasculitic involvement at the periphery. Treatment includes topical, intralesional, and/or systemic corticosteroids. Minocycline, dapsone, and more recently cyclosporin A have proved to be beneficial in some patients.

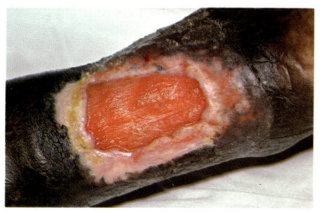

125 Pyoderma gangrenosum. This West Indian man developed a pustule over the lower leg which progressed to a tender, superficial necrotic ulcer. Note the typical purple undermined edge. The lesion persisted for months and partially responded to topical corticosteroids and minocycline. Eventually, it responded to systemic corticosteroids. No underlying disease was identified.

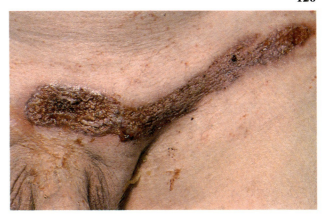

126 Pyoderma gangrenosum in the groin. This middle-aged man developed linear necrotic ulceration in his left groin, which extended rapidly despite topical and systemic corticosteroids. There was no response to minocycline, but eventually low-dose cyclosporin A was curative. He had suffered from rheumatoid arthritis for many years.

Polyarteritis nodosa

There are two forms of polyarteritis nodosa (PAN), cutaneous and systemic. Cutaneous PAN presents with a livedo pattern (**121**) dominant over the knees, thighs, and calves, with interspersed tender nodules. Rarely, there is associated neuropathy and myalgia. Prognosis is good.

The systemic form of PAN presents with a vasculitic rash (**127**), hypertension, pericarditis, abdominal symptoms, and neurological and renal disease. Investigations may reveal elevated erythrocyte sedimentation rate (ESR), low serum complement, elevated serum gammaglobulins, leucocytosis, eosinophilia, and anaemia. The involvement of medium-sized systemic arteries in the vasculitic process can often be demonstrated by arteriography, which may show characteristic aneurysms (**128**). Deep skin biopsy, or renal biopsy where there is renal involvement, shows characteristic vasculitic changes (**129**).

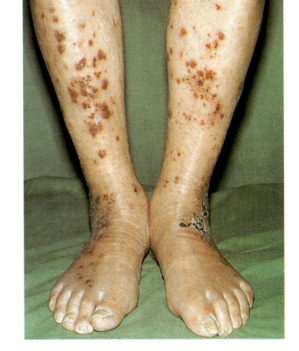

127 Polyarteritis nodosa (PAN) commonly presents with a purpuric, vasculitic eruption, as in this 70-year-old man. The rash is typically less uniform than that of leucocytoclastic vasculitis, and because PAN affects the deeper vessels of the skin, the rash may often take on a livedo appearance (see **121**). This patient had systemic PAN, with symptoms and signs suggesting a polyneuropathy, and evidence of renal failure. Despite high-dose corticosteroid therapy, he died from renal failure within 2 months of presentation.

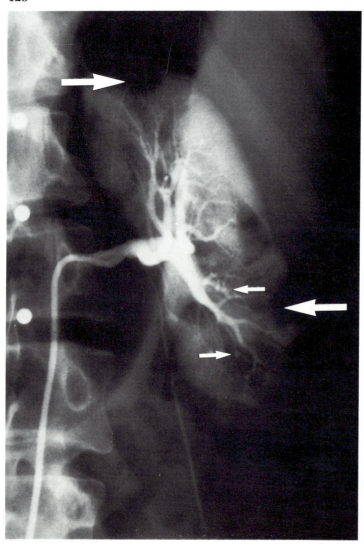

128 The systemic form of polyarteritis nodosa (PAN) commonly affects the kidney. This selective left renal arteriogram shows typical arteritic aneurysms of the intra-renal vessels (small arrows) and subcapsular areas of renal infarction (large arrows). Similar changes may occur in other organs, including the liver, the spleen, and the central and peripheral nervous system, but renal damage is the commonest cause of death in PAN.

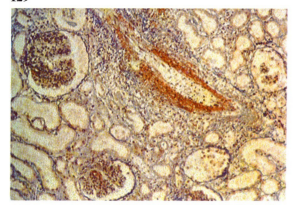

129 Renal biopsy in a patient with PAN (MSB x 118). Note the proliferative changes in the glomeruli and the fibrinoid necrosis (stained red) of the interlobular artery. The arteritic process is similar to that seen elsewhere in the body in this condition. It usually begins in the media and extends to the outer coats of the arterial wall. Necrosis and inflammatory cell infiltration follow, and may result in fibrosis and luminal thrombosis, or in aneurysm formation.

The cause of PAN is unknown, but 20–40% of patients are hepatitis B antigen positive, and it is likely that immune-complex deposition, following this and other infections, plays an important role.

Treatment is with high-dose corticosteroids, usually in combination with an immunosuppressive agent, e.g. azathioprine. The prognosis is variable. Spontaneous remission may occur, but death usually supervenes within months to years, due to renal complications.

Erythema nodosum

Erythema nodosum is primarily an inflammation of the subcutaneous fat (panniculitis), with involvement of the adjacent vasculature. It is an immunological reaction (probably Type III) elicited by various infections, drugs, and a variety of other causes (*Table 22*).

The characteristic lesions are tender, red nodules occurring on the lower legs and sometimes the forearms (**130, 131**). Some patients also have painful joints and fever. The lesions resolve in 6–8 weeks, often leaving a bruise-like appearance. Management depends on the identification and elimination of the underlying cause. Otherwise bed-rest, non-steroidal anti-inflammatory drugs, and, for reasons which are not clear, potassium iodide can help (but this should not be used for longer than 6 months).

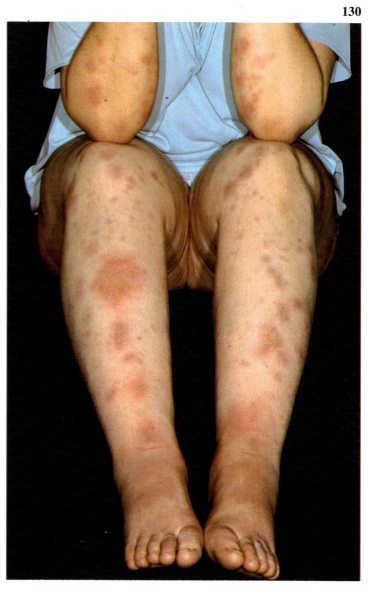

130 Erythema nodosum occurring in a classic distribution over the front of the legs and forearms. The appearance reflects the patchy inflammation of subcutaneous fat and small vessels, probably as the result of a Type III (immune complex) allergic mechanism. Erythema nodosum has many causes. This patient also had arthralgia and a mild fever, and further investigation revealed an underlying diagnosis of sarcoidosis.

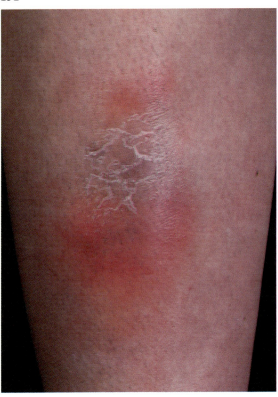

Table 22. *Some causes of erythema nodosum.*

Infections
Bacterial (e.g., streptococcal, tuberculosis, brucellosis, leprosy)
Mycoplasma
Rickettsia
Chlamydia
Viral
Fungal (e.g., coccidioidomycosis, histoplasmosis)

Drugs
(e.g., sulphonamides, contraceptive pill)

Systemic disease
(e.g. sarcoidosis, inflammatory bowel disease, Beçhet's disease)

131 Erythema nodosum. This close-up view shows a large lesion which had been present (with others) for several weeks. Dehiscence of the epidermis is not uncommon in chronic lesions, and they may gradually take on a range of appearances, becoming violaceous or assuming any of the colours of a resolving bruise. In this patient, erythema nodosum was associated with Crohn's disease.

Erythema multiforme

Erythema multiforme is also immunologically mediated, but it may be due to a combination of Type III and Type IV hypersensitivity reactions. The patient has usually reacted to an underlying antigen, e.g. herpes simplex or a drug, but other factors have occasionally been implicated (*Table 23*).

Symptoms of infection may precede the eruption, which typically takes the form of annular plaques over the palms, soles, and limbs (**132, 133**) and sometimes over the trunk (**10**). Characteristic 'target' lesions made up of two concentric plaques may blister in the centre. When combined with mucous membrane involvement, erythema multiforme is called the Stevens–Johnson syndrome (**10, 134**). Lesions in the tracheobronchial tree in such patients may lead to asphyxia, and conjunctival and corneal involvement may result in blindness. Genital ulcers may cause urinary retention and phimosis or vaginal stricture after they have healed.

Skin biopsy is distinctive, with upper dermal and perivascular inflammation and epidermal necrosis suggesting a cell-mediated pathogenesis rather than a vasculitis. However, antigens such as herpes virus

Table 23. *Some causes of erythema multiforme.*

Viral infection, e.g. herpes simplex, hepatitis, orf
Mycoplasma infection
Bacterial infections
Fungal infections, e.g. coccidioidomycosis
Parasitic infections
Drugs
Pregnancy
Malignancy and its treatment with radiotherapy
Idiopathic

have been identified in the skin lesions. Most investigations are directed towards identifying a cause, but about 50% of cases have no demonstrable provoking factor.

Treatment ideally includes removal of an identifiable cause; otherwise, it is symptomatic. In Stevens–Johnson syndrome, a multidisciplinary approach is often required. The effectiveness of systemic corticosteroids is debatable and, ideally, short-term in the acute stage. Recurrent erythema multiforme due to herpes simplex may respond to acyclovir or even to low-dose azathioprine.

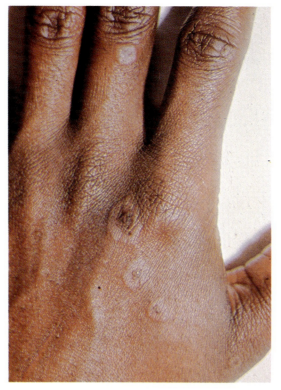
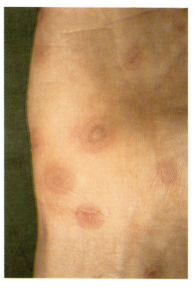

132 Erythema multiforme is a form of reactive erythema which probably involves both Type III and Type IV immunological mechanisms. Typically, it starts with a symmetrical eruption of target-like lesions on the hands and feet. These may blister centrally and they spread proximally, the extent depending on the severity of involvement. This patient is mildly affected (compare with **10**). Like erythema nodosum, erythema multiforme may have many causes; but in 50% of patients – as in this case – no cause is found.

133 Erythema multiforme is often something of a misnomer, because the lesions tend to be uniform in their character, as seen here. The concentric 'target' lesions seen in this close-up view of the hypothenar eminence are typical.

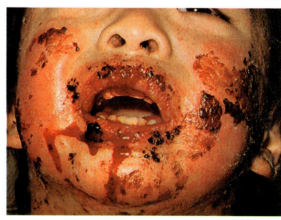

134 Stevens–Johnson syndrome is potentially fatal. In this 2-year-old Chinese boy it developed following co-trimoxazole administration.

Erythema elevatum diutinum

Erythema elevatum diutinum is a very rare form of chronic vasculitis, in which lesions are localised to extensor surfaces on hands (**135**), elbows, knees, and ankles. Characteristically, lesions are symmetrical red–brown–purple nodules and plaques which may occasionally ulcerate, but unlike those of small vessel vasculitis these lesions remain static for months. Systemic involvement is unusual, but recurrent streptococcal infection or concomitant IgA myeloma are recognised as underlying causes.

135 Erythema elevatum diutinum. This middle-aged man presented with symmetrical red–brown–purple nodules occurring on the back of his hands, elbows, and knees. Biopsy revealed a chronic vasculitis. The underlying antigen in this condition is unknown, but systemic involvement is rare. Further investigations in this patient revealed an underlying IgA myeloma.

Vasculitis with Granuloma Formation

A number of vasculitic conditions are accompanied by significant granulomatous infiltration, particularly if the course of the disease is chronic. They can thus be differentiated from 'pure' vasculitis on histological grounds.

Polymyalgia rheumatica and temporal arteritis

The relationship between polymyalgia rheumatica and temporal or giant cell arteritis is sufficiently close for the two disorders to be regarded as different manifestations of the same process. The former is more common, but arteritis can be found in 50% of patients.

Both conditions occur in the elderly, and their onset may be insidious or abrupt, with malaise, weight loss, and low-grade fever. The myalgia involves tenderness, stiffness, and aching of proximal muscles. Synovitis is common, not only in the shoulders and hips, but also in the knees, where it may be clinically apparent. Skin signs are not usually present.

Temporal arteritis is an important cause of headache in the elderly; early diagnosis and treatment are essential to remove the risk of blindness from involvement of the posterior ciliary arteries and the central retinal artery branches. Blindness in one or both eyes occurs in 30% of untreated patients. The other cerebral and coronary vessels are rarely affected. Burning and tenderness over the scalp are common symptoms, and the patient may have prominent and tender temporal arteries (**136**), but these signs are not always present.

Investigations in both conditions may reveal a normochromic anaemia, a high ESR, and raised acute-phase proteins, but leucocytosis is absent. Temporal artery biopsy reveals a necrotising patchy arteritis, with large mononuclear cell infiltration and giant cells (**137**).

Treatment of both conditions involves systemic corticosteriods; their early administration in temporal arteritis may prevent blindness. Temporal arteritis often occurs in isolation, but polymyalgia rheumatica may be a manifestation of occult malignancy, early rheumatoid arthritis, or a chronic infection such as infective endocarditis.

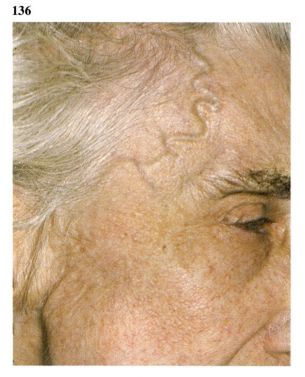

136 Temporal arteritis. This 78-year-old woman presented with severe headaches. Her right temporal artery was prominent and tender, and her ESR was grossly elevated. Biopsy confirmed the diagnosis of temporal arteritis, and she was treated immediately with systemic corticosteroids.

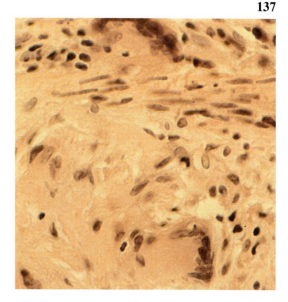

137 Temporal arteritis is also known as cranial arteritis or giant cell arteritis. It is a true panarteritis, affecting vessels of all sizes, and it is characterised histologically by granulomatous thickening of the vessel wall, with an infiltrate containing lymphocytes, epithelioid cells, and multinucleate giant cells. This close-up view of a biopsy sample is typical, showing a giant cell at the top. The arteritic changes may be patchy, so the diagnosis is not excluded by a single negative biopsy.

Rheumatoid arthritis

Rheumatoid arthritis is a common condition, affecting all races, and females more commonly than males. It is a multisystem disorder, and in addition to the characteristic arthritis (**138**), it may cause peripheral neuropathy, lung and pleural involvement, pericarditis, eye involvement, and normochromic normocytic anaemia. Many of these manifestations are the result of a granulomatous vasculitic process, which may also lead to the characteristic skin signs of the disease, including leucocytoclastic vasculitis (**116**), subcutaneous nodules (**139**), peri-ungual haemorrhage and infarction (**140**), and arterial ulcers which may be relatively minor (**141**) or major (**142**). Because of its chronicity, the disease may ultimately be complicated by amyloidosis.

Rheumatoid factor is found in most patients, especially when subcutaneous nodules are present. Rheumatoid factor is an antiglobulin, most commonly an IgM which reacts with human IgG. It is also found in up to 30% of patients with SLE, PAN, scleroderma, and dermatomyositis.

Treatment of rheumatoid arthritis may include bedrest, local therapy, systemic therapy with nonsteroidal anti-inflammatory drugs and with more potent but hazardous agents, such as gold, penicillamine, chloroquine, and corticosteroids if necessary.

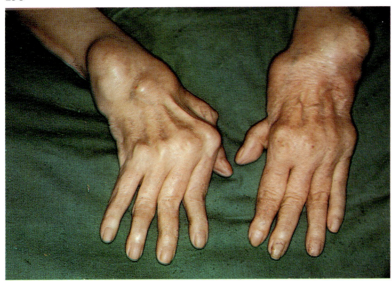

138 Severe rheumatoid arthritis results in severe deformity and disability. The appearance of these hands is typical of the long-standing disease. Note the marked ulnar deviation of the fingers, and the 'swan neck' deformity, which results from disruption of the tendons and tendon sheaths of the fingers. There is also marked muscle wasting and massive tendon sheath swelling over the dorsal surfaces of both wrists.

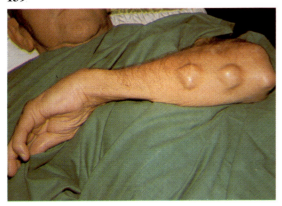

139 Rheumatoid nodules commonly present as lobulated swellings in the upper forearm and over the elbow. Histologically, rheumatoid nodules show vasculitic and granulomatous changes.

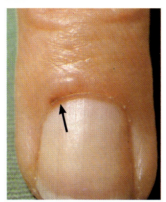 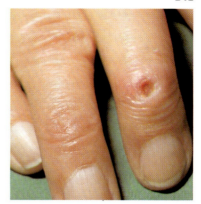

140 Vasculitic lesions around the nails occur in a number of autoimmune disorders, including rheumatoid arthritis. At this stage in development (arrow) they may be painful and tender. They may resolve or progress to become small infarcts.

141 Vasculitic lesions in the skin in rheumatoid arthritis may progress to produce ulceration, as here at the distal interphalangeal joint. Small ulcers like this commonly heal by revascularisation from the edge of the lesion, but multiple and recurrent ulceration may occur.

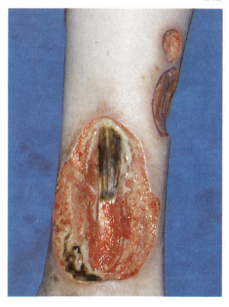

142 Massive ulceration may result from vasculitis in rheumatoid arthritis, as in this patient. Multiple, deep arterial ulcers have occurred on the legs. The largest ulcer shows clearly a mass of necrotic tissue and exposed tendons in its base. Histology confirmed an underlying vasculitis. Such ulcers are very difficult to treat, but may respond to a combination of aggressive therapy for the rheumatoid arthritis and careful nursing care. Amputation may be necessary for severely affected legs, if other therapy fails.

Granulomatous vasculitis

Granulomatous vasculitis (allergic granulomatous angiitis) is also termed the Churg–Strauss syndrome and is a rare vasculitis distinguished by adult-onset asthma, peripheral eosinophilia, and recurrent pneumonia. Patients may have hypertension, fever, weight loss, and gastrointestinal and cardiac involvement, as in PAN, but renal disease is unusual; 60% have palpable purpura, cutaneous infarction, and tender subcutaneous nodules. Pathologically, there is leucocytoclastic vasculitis with additional abundant eosinophilia and so-called flame figures. In the latter, particularly when nodules are present clinically, a granulomatous reaction pattern is also evident. High-dose corticosteroids are the drugs of choice.

Wegener's granulomatosis

Typically, the initial symptoms and signs of Wegener's granulomatosis include fever, weight loss, and fatigue, accompanied by nasorespiratory symptoms, such as rhinitis, hearing loss, and sinusitis. Only half of the patients have skin lesions, including symmetrical ulcers or papules on the extremities. As the disease progresses, it often involves the nasal septum, leading to a characteristic saddle-nose deformity (**143, 144**). Other organs involved include the eye, joints, heart, nerves, lung, and kidney. Although the cause is unknown, antineutrophil antibodies are present in most cases and are a useful diagnostic marker. Skin biopsy may reveal leucocytoclastic vasculitis and/or necrotising granulomatous vasculitis. The combination of systemic corticosteroids and cyclophosphamide is the treatment of choice, but the disease still carries a high mortality rate – especially from renal failure.

143

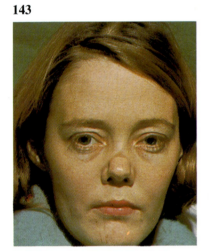

144

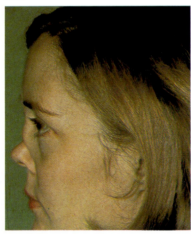

143, 144 Wegener's granulomatosis typically destroys the nasal cartilage, producing a saddle-nose deformity. At this stage, the diagnosis can usually be confirmed by nasal biopsy. Skin lesions occur in about 50% of patients, and skin biopsy may show vasculitic and granulomatous changes.

Lymphomatoid and lethal midline granulomatosis

These very rare conditions are both angiodestructive processes involving primarily the upper respiratory tract. Patients are usually males with systemic symptoms and signs resembling Wegener's granulomatosis. However, 50% have polymorphic cutaneous lesions, most commonly in the form of red to violaceous papules, plaques, and nodules. Skin anergy is often present. Skin biopsy reveals a deep angiocentric mixed inflammatory infiltrate. Recent studies have confirmed that there is a monoclonal proliferation of T-cells in both conditions, supporting the concept that these disorders should be reclassified as cutaneous T-cell lymphomas. Prognosis is poor despite immunosuppressive drugs and cytotoxic agents. At least 15% of patients develop a clear-cut large cell immunoblastic T-cell lymphoma.

7 Skin Disorders Associated with Delayed Allergic Reactions

Delayed Gell and Coombs' Type IV allergic reactions are involved in a number of skin diseases, and the two most common disorders which involve Type IV mechanisms are atopic eczema (atopic dermatitis) and contact dermatitis (contact eczema). It is important to distinguish clinically between atopic eczema and contact dermatitis.

Atopic eczema is difficult to define, because its aetiology and pathogenesis are unknown. It is an endogenous skin disease that predominantly, but not exclusively, affects young children, and it is characterised by itchy epidermal lesions. It runs a chronic and relapsing course. There is a genetic predisposition to the disease, most patients have raised circulating IgE levels, and it is commonly associated with a personal or family history of atopic disease, such as asthma and hay fever. Type I allergic mechanisms may play a role in the early stages of the disease, but – despite the continuing association with other Type I reactions – it seems likely that many later features of the disease are manifestations of Type IV delayed hypersensitivity or other abnormalities (see also page 114).

Contact dermatitis is relatively simple to define: it is an eczematous eruption produced by external agents (exogenous dermatitis). The reaction may be acute or chronic, and it may be produced by Type IV allergic mechanisms, directly by irritants, or by photosensitive reactions (allergic or non-allergic). Contact irritant dermatitis is much commoner than contact allergic dermatitis, accounting for around 80% of cases of contact dermatitis.

Contact Allergic Dermatitis

Contact allergic dermatitis is a delayed-type immunological reaction of the skin caused by an exogenous allergen. Virtually any chemical has the potential to cause this type of reaction, and the most frequent are outlined in *Table 24*. The eruption ranges from acute, weeping, crusted vesicles and bullae, which develop within 24–48 hours, to chronic, lichenified plaques. There may be a delay in the development of lesions of up to 4 days in a sensitised individual; and sensitisation takes at least 7 days. Characteristically, the lesions have angular corners, linear streaks, or sharp margins, suggesting an external source. The delayed onset of the eczema often makes the cause obscure, requiring a detailed personal and occupational history, and patch testing to identify the precipitating chemical. Moreover, contact

Table 24. *Some common allergens in contact dermatitis.*

Allergen	Sources
Nickel	Jewellery, jean studs, bra clips, tools
Balsam of Peru	Perfumes, citrus fruits
Dichromate	Cement, leather, matches
Paraphenylenediamine	Hair dyes, clothing
Rubber chemicals	Shoes, clothing, gloves
Colophony (rosin)	Sticking plaster, collodion
Neomycin	Topical medicaments
Benzocaine	Topical anaesthetics
Parabens	Preservatives in cosmetics and creams
Wool alcohols	Lanolin, cosmetics, creams
Imidazolidinyl urea	Preservative in creams and cosmetics
Formaldehyde (aqueous)	Clothing, cosmetics, glues, paper
Epoxy resin	Glues

allergic dermatitis is morphologically identical to other eczematous eruptions (see Chapter 10). Other causes of eczema and eczema-like dermatoses should be excluded, including superficial fungal infections. Therapy includes topical corticosteroids, but prevention by avoidance of the allergen is the best solution.

Distribution of lesions in contact allergic dermatitis

The distribution pattern of eczema can often suggest an exogenous allergen. The head and neck are frequent sites when the allergens occur in cosmetics, but the links are not always obvious. Eczema of the eyelids is almost always a contact dermatitis and may be due to nail varnish, for example. Permanent wave lotion and hair dyes may produce scalp and facial eczema in clients and hand eczema in hairdressers. An eruption involving the exposed skin of the head, neck, and arms suggests a photoallergic reaction (Chapter 8) or an airborne contact dermatitis. The dorsum of the hands is the most common site of contact allergy from industrial chemicals, e.g. cutting oils. The dorsum of the foot, however, suggests rubber compounds or tanning agents in shoes (**8**). Involvement of the earlobes, neck, and wrists suggests the possibility of nickel allergy from jewellery worn at these sites (this affects 10% of all Western women). A worsening dermatitis in any location suggests an allergic reaction to the topical medication used to treat the original eruption. Interestingly, it has been recently recognised that some patients can develop contact allergic dermatitis to topical corticosteroids.

Often, neither the location nor the timing point to the cause of contact allergic dermatitis, and only a detailed history and a positive patch test make it possible to identify the occult allergen.

Pathogenesis of contact allergic dermatitis

Contact allergic dermatitis is a good example of a cell-mediated Type IV delayed immunological reaction. There are two phases in its pathogenesis. The first is sensitisation, during which the individual becomes allergic to the chemical. This takes about 7 days and probably occurs in the regional lymph node producing memory, effector, and suppressor T-lymphocytes. The second phase, elicitation, occurs over 1–2 days with continued or repeated exposure to the allergen and results in contact allergic dermatitis. The causative chemical, the hapten, is usually a compound of low molecular weight (less than 500 daltons). It must be able to penetrate the stratum corneum and it then binds to a carrier protein, which is probably on the surface of the Langerhans cells. The antigen is then processed and re-expressed to the cell surface with the HLA DR receptor site for presentation to the T-helper (CD4) lymphocytes (see Chapter 2). Contact allergic dermatitis represents a balance between elicitation and suppression, with the reaction ultimately extinguished by suppressor mechanisms, which are thought to include suppressor T-cells and serum factors.

Common allergens

Poison ivy, poison oak, and poison sumac (all members of the genus *Rhus*) are the most frequent causes of contact allergic dermatitis in the USA (**7**). Approximately 50% of the adult population is sensitive. The allergen (an oleoresin – urushiol) is found in the sap of these plants. Cross reactivity occurs with other related plants, e.g. the cashew, Japanese lacquer, mango, and masking nut trees; and those working with products from these trees (shelling cashew nuts, or peeling mangoes) may develop contact dermatitis of the hands.

Nickel sensitivity occurs in 10% of all females (**145–148**), but is much rarer in men. Where it is suspected, the presence of nickel in metal items can be confirmed by the dimethyl–glyoxime spot test. Avoidance is the only means of preventing inflammation, and sources of contact include jewellery, watch bands, belt buckles, scissors, door handles, and screws in orthopaedic implants. In highly sensitive individuals, ingested nickel from cooking utensils may play a role in aggravating dermatitis – especially pompholyx – and in hindering its control.

Paraphenylenediamine is a common colouring agent used in permanent hair dyes and fur coats. It can therefore affect the scalp and face (**11, 149**), and the hands.

Iatrogenic contact allergic dermatitis can be caused by chloramphenicol (**192**), atropine, neomycin, or ethylenediamine.

Many other allergens may also cause allergic contact dermatitis (**8, 150–160**).

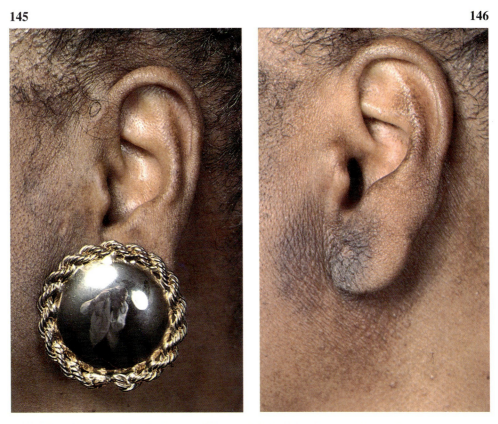

145, 146 Contact allergic dermatitis to nickel. This affects 10% of European women. Nickel is a commonly used metal, found in jewellery such as earrings, necklaces, bracelets, and rings. Nickel contained in the large earring (**145**) gave rise to eczema of the ear lobe and facial skin (**146**) in this young woman.

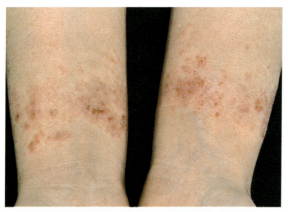

147 Nickel contact allergy. A severe dermatitis has developed due to a Type IV hypersensitivity reaction to nickel in bracelets worn on both the wrists of this young woman. Nickel is also commonly found in bra clips and studs on jeans.

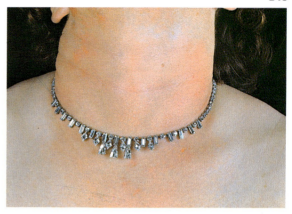

148 Nickel contact allergy. Another example, showing a reaction to nickel in a necklace, with the resulting dermatitis affecting the neck. Note the widespread involvement, aggravated by scratching and rubbing.

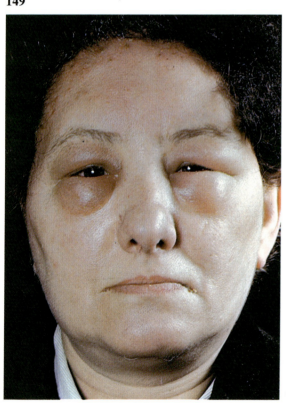

149 Facial dermatitis. This is an example of contact allergic dermatitis affecting the face. This patient had both pruritus and facial oedema. The oedema was prominent, especially around her eyes, but her history revealed that the eruption was chronic and not intermittent, which ruled out angioedema as the cause. Her dermatitis developed following the use of hair dye. On examination, she had eczematous changes all over the scalp; and patch testing confirmed a positive reaction to paraphenylenediamine, which is present in black hair dyes (see also **11**).

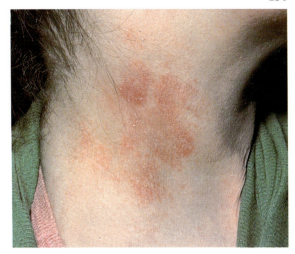

150 Nail varnish contact allergy. This woman had characteristic localised dermatitis on her neck, due to the transfer of nail varnish by repeated skin contact – she scratched her neck with her nails as a nervous mannerism.

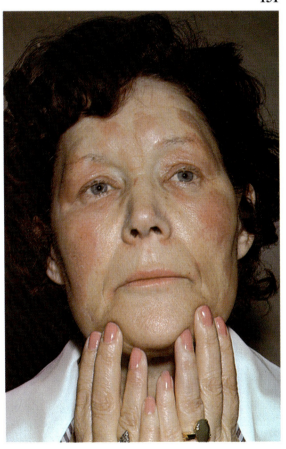

151 Facial dermatitis. This middle-aged lady developed a contact allergic dermatitis to face cream. Patch testing confirmed a Type IV hypersensitivity reaction to lanolin, which is commonly found in many cosmetic creams.

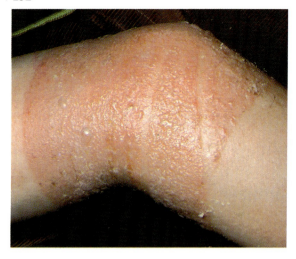

152 Rubber contact allergy. This 28-year-old lady developed an acute erythematous vesicular dermatitis as a consequence of Type IV hypersensitivity to rubber in an elasticated bandage. Rubber allergy was confirmed by patch testing.

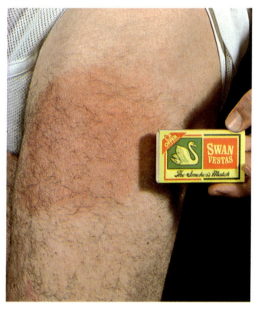

153 Contact allergy to phosphorus sequisulphide. This 50-year-old man had dermatitis of his face, hands, and right thigh, which resulted from hypersensitivity to the chemical in red-tipped matches. Note the relationship of the thigh dermatitis to the area of the trouser pocket in which he carried his matches. Typically, these patients react to the slightest exposure.

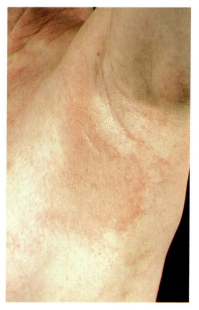

154 Axillary dermatitis. This distribution is often a clue to a contact allergy. Surprisingly, in this case the culprit was wool alcohols in a body lotion. Probably the commonest cause is allergy to preservatives in underarm deodorants.

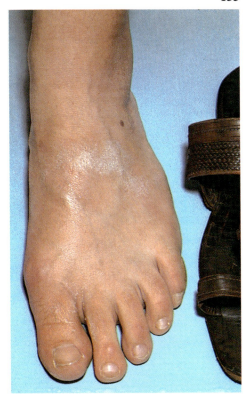

155 Sandal dermatitis. The pattern shown here suggests a contact allergy. This lady developed Type IV hypersensitivity to chromate, which is used as a tanning agent in curing leather (see also **8**).

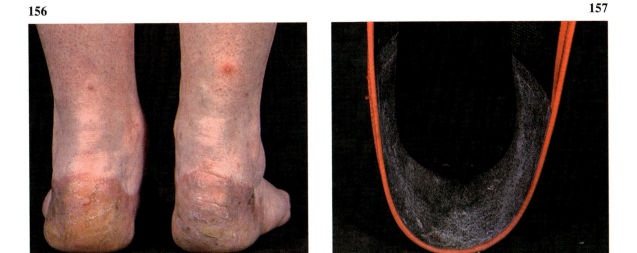

156, 157 Shoe dermatitis. The dermatitis affects predominantly the heels (**156**) of this middle-aged man, and patch testing revealed a positive reaction to the rubber glue used as an adhesive in the lining of his shoes (**157**). These chemicals are leached out by sweat.

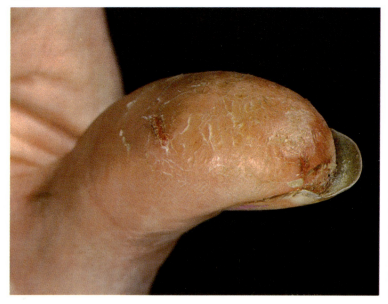

158 Garlic dermatitis. This left-handed cook developed dermatitis on the tips of her right thumb and index finger, due to repeated contact with garlic. Other foods which can cause contact allergic dermatitis include carrot, parsnip, parsley, celery, various spices, and mango.

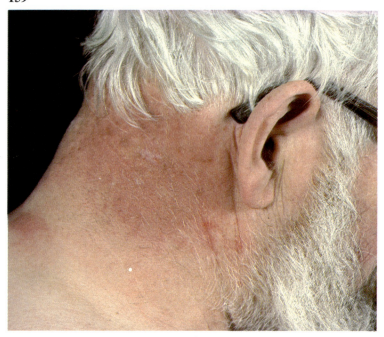

159 Caterpillar dermatitis. Many caterpillars are venomous due to setae, which are hair-like, sometimes hollow, spiny structures present on the surface at most stages of their development. The venoms contain inflammatory mediators, which can result in papules, weals, and eczematisation 6–12 hours after contact. The setae are often blown into the air from the caterpillars, and they may land in large quantities on exposed sites, as shown on this man's neck. The rash can persist as a dermatitis for up to several weeks. Atopic individuals are particularly susceptible to severe reactions.

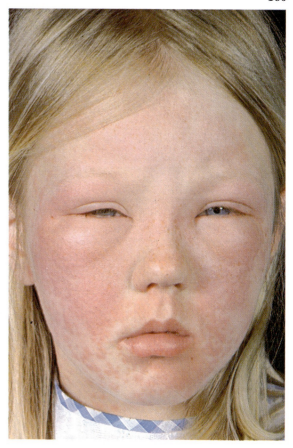

160 Severe caterpillar dermatitis caused by the brown tail moth. The brown tail moth is a cosmopolitan genus, and some species are found in southern England and across Europe as far as the Caucasus. It has also been introduced into North America. An immunological mechanism is probably involved in this reaction, and it is likely that both Type I and Type IV hypersensitivity reactions play a role.

Patch testing

Patch testing is a simple procedure but to be meaningful it must be properly performed and interpreted (see Chapter 3 and **161–164**). Figures vary in different centres, but even with careful selection, less than half the patients tested will have a positive result and only 50% of the positive results will be relevant to the current problem. Patch testing is best avoided in pregnancy, but there are no other contra-indications to its use. Active sensitisation to test allergens is rare.

Patch testing is discussed in more detail in Chapter 3.

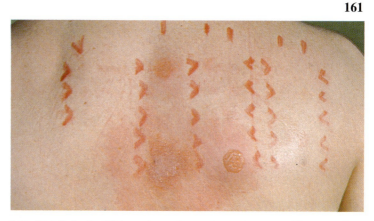

161 Patch tests. This patient shows very strong positive reactions to three test substances following a 48-hour application of the patch test battery recommended by the International Contact Dermatitis Research Group. Labelling with a felt-tipped pen ensures that the allergens can be recognised. Such a result should alert the investigator to a possible 'angry back' syndrome – i.e. to false positive results (see Chapter 3). This can be excluded by testing each allergen separately.

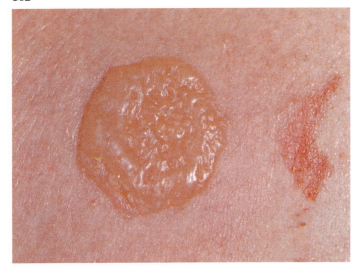

162 Positive patch test. This result shows a +++ reaction to rubber mix, with widespread erythema and intense vesiculation (see *Table 7*).

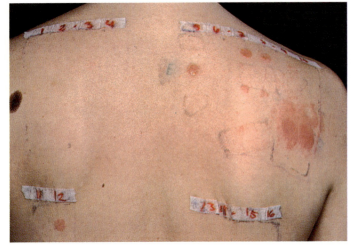
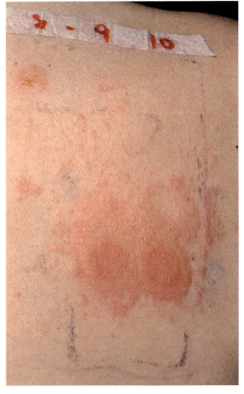

163, 164 Contact allergy to topical corticosteroids. This young woman demonstrated intense positive patch tests to several topical corticosteroids. This is a recently recognised problem, which can be easily overlooked and may be responsible for apparent resistance to treatment. Confirmation is simple: the corticosteroid can be tested on a normal area of skin in an open manner or added to a standard patch test battery.

Management

Avoidance of the allergen is the key to treatment, but where allergen avoidance is impossible, or where symptoms persist despite avoidance, the treatment of contact allergic dermatitis is similar to that of other forms of eczema (see Chapter 11).

Contact Irritant Dermatitis

Contact irritant dermatitis represents 80% of all contact-related dermatoses. Like allergic reactions it may be acute or chronic, and the clinical and pathological features of contact allergic and irritant dermatitis can be identified (**165**). The response to irritants usually peaks at 24–48 hours, with gradual resolution within hours or even several days. An exception is sodium lauryl sulphate which reacts later; so the initial 48-hour reading on patch testing is often falsely negative, and a further reading should be made 2–8 hours after removal of the patch.

Irritants vary in their chemical composition and potential for skin damage. Strong irritants, such as wet cement, can produce dermatitis on initial contact, but milder forms, such as detergents and urine (**166**), require prolonged exposure. Physical factors, such as friction, trauma, and humidity, as well as age, co-existent atopy, and skin site, are important. It is often the additive effect of several factors which triggers the dermatitis.

Management is mainly by prevention and avoidance of the offending agent through proper skin care and protection. In an occupational setting this may involve protective clothing, such as shields, goggles, or gloves. Medical treatment – where required – is similar to that for other forms of eczema (see Chapter 11).

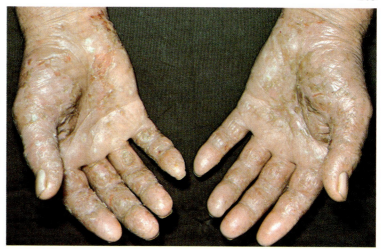

165 Contact irritant dermatitis. This middle-aged man has been exposed to irritant chemicals, such as cutting oils, at work for several years. This has resulted in severe hand dermatitis, which has impetiginised and required him to take time off work. Culprit substances are usually easily identified, but sometimes a factory visit and further detective work are necessary.

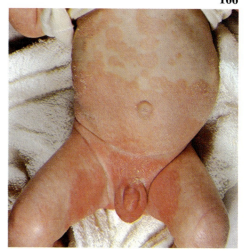

166 Nappy (diaper) dermatitis. This is a common problem and is usually an irritant contact dermatitis due to ammonia produced by urea-splitting bacteria aggravated by waterproof plastic pants. It is not usually a manifestation of atopic eczema. Note the sparing of the skin folds, suggesting an exogenous cause. Superinfection with *Candida albicans* is common and may lead to satellite papules.

Photoallergy

Photoallergy is most frequently produced by sunscreen components, such as *para*-aminobenzoic acid and its esters, by benzophenones, and by fragrance additives in cosmetics, e.g. musk ambrette and methylcoumarin. The eruption is eczematous and limited to sun-exposed areas (see Chapter 8). A suspected diagnosis of photocontact allergy can be confirmed by photopatch testing (see Chapter 3).

Atopic Eczema and Immune Mechanisms

Atopic eczema is a common disorder, with a prevalence of over 5% in children, but its pathogenesis is still unclear. However, there is strong evidence that both IgE-mediated immediate and Type IV late phase reactions play a major role in the development of the disorder. In addition, a consistent defect in T-lymphocyte suppressor function has also been documented. Perhaps suppression of IgE synthesis is less efficient in atopic than in normal individuals. Moreover, there is a hyper-releasability of histamine by blood basophils associated with an elevated phosphodiesterease activity. Over the years there have been attempts to implicate food allergies, but these do not suggest that food antigens play a major role in most patients (see Chapter 9). More recent work has, however, suggested that aeroallergens, such as house dust mite excreta, may play a role. Many patients with atopic eczema have both positive Type I and positive Type IV skin tests to dust mite allergen, and several other studies have supported the idea that aeroallergens may cause eczematous reactions in patients with atopic eczema. Atopic eczema is reviewed in more detail in Chapter 10.

Auto-eczematisation

Auto-eczematisation (autosensitisation dermatitis) is dissemination of a previously localised area of chronic eczema to distant parts of the skin. This phenomenon often occurs suddenly and may occur with many types of eczema, including, for example, stasis or varicose eczema. The pathogenesis is a mystery, but a cell-mediated (Type IV) autoimmune mechanism has been suggested. A generalised hyperirritable skin is another possibility. Treatment depends on control of the original site of chronic eczema, with concomitant treatment of the distal site.

Dermatitis occurring as an allergic reaction (an *id* reaction) to a fungal infection elsewhere on the skin is termed a dermatophytid (**167**). The criteria for diagnosis consist of a dermal fungal infection, e.g. tinea pedis, distant eczema, such as pompholyx on one palm devoid of fungus, a positive skin test to fungal antigen, and resolution of the *id* reaction following treatment of the fungal infection. This clinical sequence is similar to that of auto-eczematisation.

167

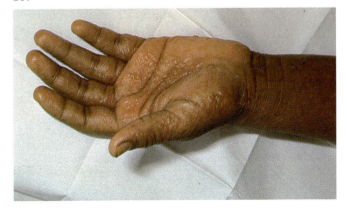

167 Pompholyx. This patient's eruption on the palm represents an *id* reaction (auto-eczematisation). It is associated with a fungal infection of the toe webs and sole of the foot. No fungus was found in scrapings of the hand, but the pompholyx resolved when the fungal infection was successfully treated with griseofulvin.

Granulomas

Granulomas are formed in the dermis where cell-mediated immunity fails to eliminate antigen. Foreign body granulomas occur because a material remains undigested. Immunological granulomas require the persistence of antigen, but the response is augmented by a cell-mediated immune reaction (Type IV). Lymphokines released by T-lymphocytes sensitised to the antigen cause macrophages to recruit and differentiate into epithelioid cells and multinuclear giant cells. These cells subsequently release other cytokines which influence inflammatory events.

Granulomatous reactions in the skin arise when infectious organisms cannot be destroyed, e.g. in tertiary syphilis (**168**), mycobacterial infections (**169, 170**), leishmaniasis (**171**), or when a chemical cannot be eliminated, e.g. zirconium, beryllium, or mercuric sulphide (**172**). Similar reactions are also seen in persisting inflammation of undetermined cause, e.g. rosacea, granuloma annulare (**15**), sarcoidosis (**173, 174**), and various subtypes of panniculitis.

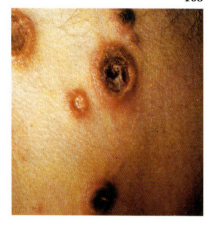

168 Tertiary syphilis, with multiple gummatous ulcers of the chest wall. Histologically, these lesions are granulomas. Delayed hypersensitivity (Type IV) reactions are undoubtedly involved in their genesis, but the underlying cause is chronic infection with *Treponema pallidum*.

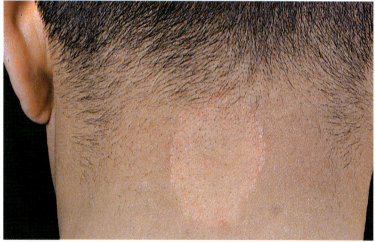

169 Leprosy. This Asian man presented with a hypopigemented patch on the back of his neck. On examination this was found to be anaesthetic. The lesion represents an early stage of tuberculoid leprosy. Histologically, the lesion shows a granulomatous reaction, especially around nerves. This form of leprosy represents a predominantly Type IV reaction to persisting infection with *Mycobacterium leprae*.

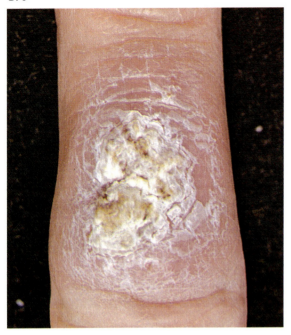

170 Fish tank granuloma. This middle-aged lady kept tropical fish and regularly cleaned out their tanks with her bare hands. This single lesion represents an infection with *Mycobacterium marinium* (*balnei*), an organism which infects fish. The lesions are often chronic, though they may resolve spontaneously and can, if necessary, be treated with antimicrobial drugs. The lesions result largely from a Type IV granulomatous reaction to the infection.

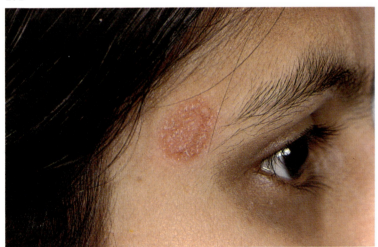

171 Cutaneous leishmaniasis. This lesion on the face of a lady from Western India resulted from infection with *Leishmania tropica*. This parasite often produces dry, single lesions, which represent a granulomatous response to the initial infection. The lesions may heal spontaneously, and may sometimes be treated by cryotherapy, but systemic therapy with antimony salts is often required for definitive treatment.

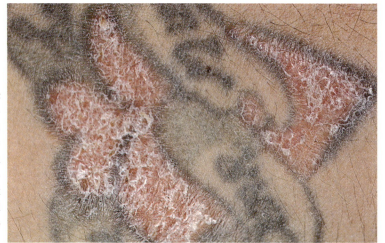

172 Granulomatous contact allergic dermatitis. This young man complained of scaling and pruritus in the red portions of a tattoo on his forearm. The appearance results from a Type IV reaction to mercuric sulphide (cinnabar), used as a pigment in the tattoo. Sometimes lichenoid reactions may result from exposure to this compound.

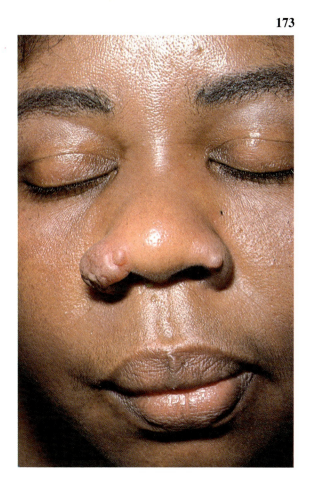

173 Sarcoidosis is a multisystem disorder which may present in many different ways, and has several different dermatological manifestations. Afro-Caribbean individuals are particularly susceptible to the disease. This young woman shows the typical distribution of cutaneous granulomas in sarcoidosis. They affect the nostrils, ear lobes, and the nape of the neck. The aetiology is unknown, but histologically the granulomas are discrete and not inflamed – unlike those seen in tuberculosis.

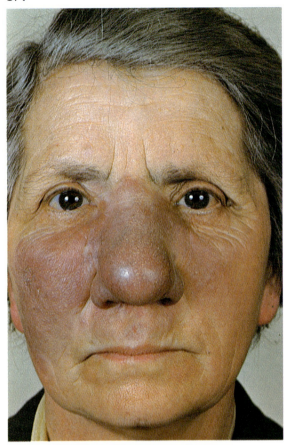

174 Lupus pernio in sarcoidosis. This 65-year-old lady has sarcoidosis affecting her nose and cheek, presenting with a typical violaceous swelling. On further investigation, there was evidence of multi-system involvement with gross bilateral hilar lymphadenopathy and parenchymal lung disease. Treatment with systemic corticosteroids had beneficial effects on her lung disease and her cutaneous lesions.

8 Photosensitivity and Photoallergy

Light has a number of important beneficial and deleterious effects on the skin in normal individuals, and some genetic and acquired disorders lead to the risk of additional damaging effects. Patients whose underlying condition renders them particularly susceptible to the effects of light are said to suffer from photosensitivity – the term is used generically, and without any implication as to the underlying mechanism. The major effects of light of different wavelengths are shown in **175** and the wide range of photosensitivity dermatoses is summarised in *Table 25*.

175

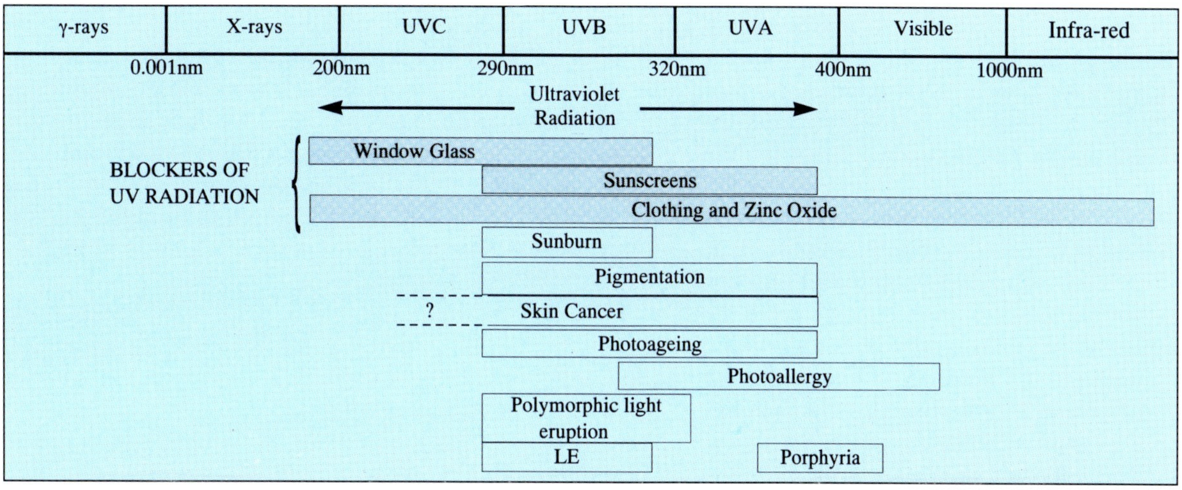

γ-rays	X-rays	UVC	UVB	UVA	Visible	Infra-red
0.001nm		200nm	290nm	320nm	400nm	1000nm

Ultraviolet Radiation

BLOCKERS OF UV RADIATION:
- Window Glass
- Sunscreens
- Clothing and Zinc Oxide

Effects:
- Sunburn
- Pigmentation
- Skin Cancer (?)
- Photoageing
- Photoallergy
- Polymorphic light eruption
- LE
- Porphyria

175 Dermatoses and photobiology. Photobiology is the study of the effects of non-ionising radiation on biological systems. Radiation is described in terms of wavelength, measured in nanometers (1 nm = 10^{-9} m). The spectrum of non-ionising radiation occupies the range of wavelengths from approximately 200 nm at the short end to radio waves (> 5,000 nm) at the long end. The ultraviolet (UV) radiation spectrum is subdivided into three parts. The C spectrum (UVC, 1–290 nm) does not penetrate the ozone layer and (at present) is irrelevant to skin disorders. The B spectrum (UVB, 290–320 nm) cause sunburn and are effectively screened out by glass. The A spectrum (UVA, 320–400 nm) is long UV light which ages and tans the skin. The wavelengths which have effects on various photosensitive dermatoses are shown here.

Table 25. *Classification of photosensitive dermatoses.*

Acute	*Exogenous chemical*
Sunburn (**176**)	Phototoxic and photoallergic reactions (**179, 180, 182–185, 197**)
Idiopathic	
Polymorphous light eruption (**177, 178**)	*Degenerative/Neoplastic*
Actinic prurigo	Solar keratoses/Squamous cell carcinoma
Chronic actinic dermatitis (**179, 180**) /Actinic reticuloid (**181**)	Basal cell carcinoma
Solar urticaria	Melanoma
	Photoageing
Photoaggravated dermatosis	*Genetic/Metabolic*
Lupus erythematosus (**186**)	Xeroderma pigmentosum
Dermatomyositis	Rothmund–Thomson syndrome
Darier's disease	Cockayne's syndrome
Acne rosacea	Bloom's syndrome
Herpes simplex	Porphyrias
Vitiligo	Hartnup disease

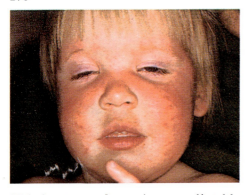

176 Acute sunburn is a predictable response to overexposure to sun, especially in fair-skinned people. This infant shows a typical appearance. Note the protection of the upper eyelids and forehead (beneath the hair) and of the nasolabial folds (in the shadow of the nose). Acute sunburn usually heals without scarring or other complications, but it leads to an increased risk of malignant melanoma; and repeated episodes of sunburn lead to premature ageing of the skin and an increased risk of basal cell and squamous cell carcinoma. It is important for everyone, of all age groups, to minimise the risk of sunburn by limiting sun exposure and using appropriate sunscreens.

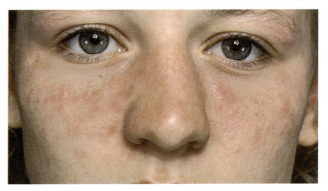

177 Polymorphous light eruption. This boy develops itchy erythematous papules over the cheek, which persist throughout the summer but fade in winter. The mechanism of this reaction – the commonest form of 'sun allergy' – is not known, but it is provoked by UVB light in the sunburn range. The reaction commonly occurs on the face and arms, but may also appear in other sun-exposed areas. It may develop at any time from 2 hours to 5 days after sun exposure – most commonly it appears within 24 hours.

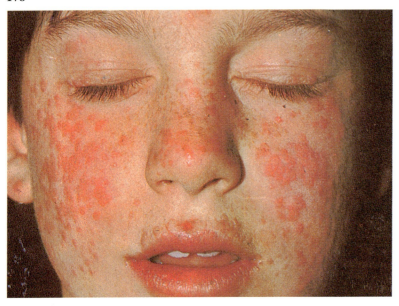

178 Hydroa vacciniforme is a form of polymorphous light eruption in which umbilicated vesicles develop, which resemble the rash of smallpox. The vesicles most commonly appear on the face, ears, chest, and back of the hands; and they may rupture and heal with scarring. As with other polymorphous light eruptions, the pathogenic mechanism in hydroa vacciniforme is obscure, but the condition tends to improve after puberty. Avoiding the sun and using sunscreens may prevent the problem, but topical corticosteroids and antimalarial drugs may be needed in severe cases.

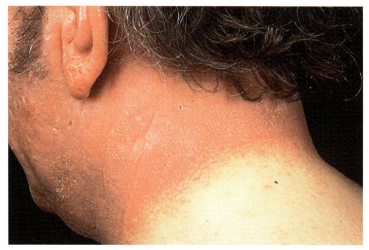

179 Chronic actinic dermatitis (photosensitive eczema) is a severe eczematous reaction which is limited to light-exposed areas. In this case, the cause was unknown and prevention of exposure to light was the major preventive measure. In many cases, however, a similar reaction may result from photosensitising drug therapy. A wide range of drugs is involved, including tetracyclines, thiazides, phenothiazines, sulphonamides, and sulphonylureas.

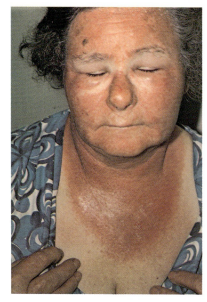

180 Chronic actinic dermatitis. In this patient, also, the cause was unknown. Note the sparing of areas not exposed to light (on the trunk), and areas that were shaded, around the eyes (by glasses) and beneath the nose.

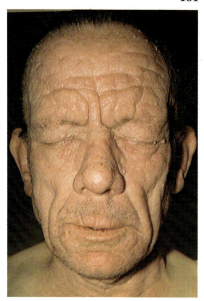

181 Actinic reticuloid of the face. There is a severe, confluent, oedematous dermatitis of light-exposed areas. The condition tends to occur in older men with pre-existing dermatitis: it probably represents a combination of chronic actinic dermatitis with the pre-existing disorder. The term 'reticuloid' refers to the histology of this condition, which may give the impression of a reticulosis to the inexperienced microscopist.

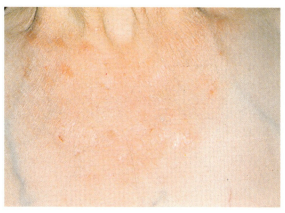

182 Phototoxic drug reaction resulting from systemic therapy. This elderly lady developed an erythematous reaction on the upper chest following exposure to the sun. Unlike the reaction seen in the patient in **180**, however, this was clearly related to the thiazide therapy which she was receiving for congestive cardiac failure. The V-neck distribution is characteristic of a photosensitive eruption.

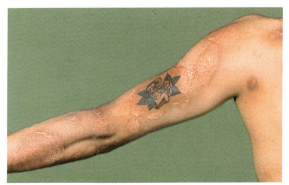

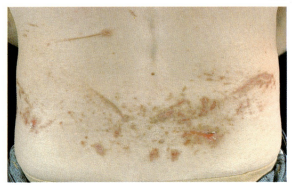

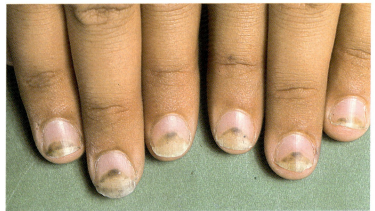

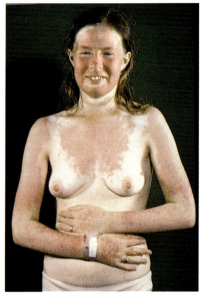

183 Phototoxic drug eruption resulting from topical therapy. This 17-year-old developed a severe eruption following treatment of his psoriasis with topical dithranol, followed by UV light.

184 Photosensitive onycholysis. This young lady returned from a Mediterranean holiday complaining of painful fingernails. She had completed a course of dimethylchlortetracycline therapy while on holiday, and it is likely that the drug provoked a phototoxic reaction. In her case, this was limited to the nail changes seen here, but associated skin changes commonly occur (see **197**).

185 Phytophotodermatitis most commonly presents with irregular streaks of erythema and hyperpigmentation occuring on the light-exposed parts of the body. On careful questioning, the patient usually gives a history of prior contact with a sensitising plant. This young man's skin had been exposed to giant hogweed. Several plant families contain substances which may induce photosensitivity in the skin, including cow parsley, hogweed, rue, and bergamot. The sensitivity results from contact with psoralen compounds within the plants. Bergapten (the active ingredient in oil of bergamot) and other furo-coumarins are also found in some perfumes. When photodermatitis results from perfume use, it is usually seen at the exposed sites of perfume application – commonly the sides of the neck.

186 Photosensitivity in systemic lupus erythematosus (SLE) is a common skin manifestation of the disease, and photosensitivity also occurs in other forms of lupus erythematosus (see Chapter 5). The involvement of light-exposed areas is obvious in this young woman. At first sight she might be thought to have severe sunburn, but the eruption followed a relatively short period of light exposure and persisted for much longer than sunburn. It is essential that patients with all forms of LE are advised on light avoidance and the use of adequate sunscreens.

Drugs and Photosensitivity

Drug-induced photosensitivity is due to the interaction of radiation and an exogenous substance in the skin. The term 'drug' in this instance is used in a very broad context, since many exogenous chromophores or photosensitisers are not therapeutic agents. All these agents have an absorption spectrum within the solar spectrum, almost always in the UVA range, but occasionally in the UVB or visible ranges.

Mechanistically, two major subtypes of reactions occur, phototoxic and photoallergic:

- A *phototoxic* reaction results in direct toxic cellular changes and skin pathology. Phototoxic reactions due to drugs often resemble exaggerated sunburn, but many different appearances may result.
- A *photoallergic* reaction is the result of photochemical production of an allergen (photoallergen), which triggers an immune response resulting in skin pathology.

The main features of the two subtypes and the drugs commonly involved are summarised in *Tables 26* and *27*. A further subclassification is usually made, based on the route of exposure of the exogenous chromophore – photocontact versus photoingestant dermatitis (systemic photosensitivity). In the clinical setting it can be difficult to distinguish between phototoxic and photoallergic reactions.

Table 26. *Features of phototoxic and photoallergic reactions.*

	Phototoxic	*Photoallergic*
Incidence	Common	Uncommon
Clinical features	Erythema and oedema Bullous Eczematous Urticarial Papular Pigmented Lichenoid Pseudoporphyria	Eczematous (erythroderma)
Onset after exposure	4–8 hours	12–24 hours
Rash occurs away from exposure site	No	Yes
Following first exposure	Can produce reaction	No reaction unless previous sensitisation period of days to months
Type of drug: topical systemic	 + +++	 +++ +
Drug dosage	Dose related	Dose independent
Immunological mechanism	None	T-cell-mediated (Type IV)

Table 27. *Drugs commonly implicated in photosensitivity reactions.*

	Phototoxic	*Photoallergic*
Topical	Coal tar derivatives, e.g. dithranol Psoralens Furocoumarins	Halogenated salicylamides
Systemic	Demeclocycline Doxycycline Chlorpromazine (occasionally)	Phenothiazines Sulphonamides Griseofulvin

Differential Diagnosis

The diagnosis of photosensitive reactions is based on the history of exposure to known phototoxic or photoallergic agents and, in the case of systemic agents, can be confirmed by phototesting (Chapter 3). The investigation is difficult and should be carried out only in specialist centres. The absence of a positive result on phototesting does not rule out the diagnosis, as the artificial radiation used is not identical to sunlight. Phototoxic contact reactions occur primarily from furocoumarins or psoralens in plants and fragrances. Photopatch testing is contraindicated in these cases, as it can result in severe blistering reactions.

A source of possible confusion in diagnosis is airborne allergic contact dermatitis. Allergy to caterpillar hairs (**159, 160**) or to pollen from plants of the *Compositae* family may give rise to contact dermatitis in exposed areas. Differential diagnosis may be difficult as both occur out of doors, but airborne allergic contact dermatitis does not require sunlight, and it also affects sites which sunlight is less likely to reach, such as behind the ears and under the chin.

Management

In most photosensitive patients, UV avoidance and/or discontinuance of the offending agent should result in resolution of the skin eruption, although persistent reactions to systemic agents have been reported, but rarely. Patients with conditions such as lupus erythematosus which are associated with photosensitivity should always be advised to avoid excessive light exposure and to use appropriate sunscreens.

9 Allergy to Drugs and Food

Drug therapy can induce a wide range of adverse reactions in the skin; indeed, drug-induced rashes are the commonest side effect of many drugs. Although the mechanisms of many of these reactions are unclear, the relationship between cause and effect is often obvious, the reactions are potentially repeatable in the same patient, and usually occur in at least some other patients receiving the same drug. Probably only about 10% of adverse drug reactions result from truly allergic mechanisms – the remainder are due to non-allergic causes – but it is generally recognised that any drug therapy carries at least a potential hazard of dermatological complications.

By contrast, the potential dermatological and other hazards of allergy or idiosyncrasy to food are much less generally agreed. Few would doubt that some foods and food additives play a causative role in some cases of urticaria or angioedema, but there is much more debate about the possible role of food in the genesis of eczema and other skin disorders – and the debate cannot be firmly resolved in the absence of agreed diagnostic procedures.

In practice, while the avoidance of specific drugs will prevent drug-induced skin disorders, the avoidance of specific foods rarely has a significant effect on the course of dermatological disorders. Nevertheless, it is wise to remember that drugs are simply a sub-group of ingested substances – albeit one which has been selected for known biological activity. It must remain likely that substances ingested in food are capable of generating at least some of the reactions which can be provoked by drug therapy; and where allergic mechanisms are involved, minute quantities of allergen can be sufficient to generate a substantial response. From first principles, it is probable that food substances – especially proteins – may be responsible for some dermatological problems in some patients, though the clinical evidence for this is still very difficult to elicit.

In this chapter we look first at drug-induced reactions in the skin and then at reactions to food; but this division may be somewhat artificial. Many of the manifestations of adverse reactions to drugs – especially those with allergic mechanisms – may yet prove also to result from adverse reactions to food or other ingested substances.

Drug Reactions in the Skin

Adverse drug reactions may result from a wide range of causes, and can be divided into three main groups:

- Non-allergic causes.
- Idiosyncratic causes.
- Allergic causes.

Non-allergic causes

Non-allergic causes are the commonest group of adverse drug reactions and may produce a wide range of manifestations (*Table 28*). Most non-allergic drug reactions can be prevented by rigid adherence to recommended drug dosage, by considering and avoiding interactions with other drugs or disease states, and by careful clinical monitoring of therapy.

Table 28. *Non-allergic causes of drug reactions in the skin.*

- *Drug overdose* or *toxicity from impaired elimination* is usually an acute phenomenon, while *intolerance* is an increased individual susceptibility to the known pharmacological effects of the drug. Dermatological consequences are not usually a major factor in these reactions.
- *Side effects* which result from known pharmacological actions of therapy may result in dermatological abnormalities. A good example is the appearance of striae and other dermatological changes in patients receiving long-term systemic or topical corticosteriod therapy.
- *Secondary effects* are an indirect result of drug action. For example, female patients on broad-spectrum antibiotic therapy often develop vaginal and vulval cardidiasis as a result of changes in microbiological flora; and oral contraceptive therapy can result in similar changes through changes in vaginal pH.
- *Teratogenicity*, such as that resulting from therapy during pregnancy with retinoids (such as etretinate), is not thought to be immunologically mediated, and skin manifestations are usually a minor part of the problem of teratogenicity.
- *Drug interactions* may lead to important systemic manifestations. Some are visible in the skin, e.g. the ecchymoses which follow the displacement of coumarin anticoagulants from plasma-binding sites by other drugs; but allergic mechanisms are not involved.

Idiosyncratic causes

Idiosyncratic reactions to drugs are unpredictable, rare, and often severe. They are not directly related to the known pharmacological activity of the drug, and their mechanisms are poorly understood. The reactions are not thought to be 'allergic', as the drug does not act as an antigen. Though the end result may closely resemble an allergic reaction, the mechanisms involved are probably 'chemical' rather than immunological in nature. They may often be a reflection of an unusual isolated metabolic abnormality in the patient receiving the drug. Dermatological examples of idiosyncratic reactions include patients who develop stomatitis when treated with methotrexate, and the hepatotoxicity which occurs in some patients treated with the antifungal drug ketoconazole.

Allergic causes

True allergic drug reactions are responses in which the drug acts as an allergen and induces a hypersensitivity state by one or more known immunological mechanism. Examples of truly allergic skin reactions include:

- Type I – urticaria or angioedema resulting from penicillin and related penicilloyl drugs.
- Type II – 'cocktail' purpura from quinine water; purpura associated with penicillin- or methyldopa-induced haemolytic anaemia.
- Type III – vasculitic reactions resulting from a wide range of drugs, including penicillins, sulphonamides, thiouracils, phenytoin, salicylic acid, streptomycin, and cholecystograhic dyes.
- Type IV – contact dermatitis in nursing or medical staff resulting from contact with injectable penicillin.

A number of clinical criteria may suggest the diagnosis of an allergic reaction (*Tables 29* and *30*).

Allergic drug reactions may be generalised, and the most serious immediate consequence is gross angioedema and anaphylaxis. Some drugs may lead to the development of a chronic immune disorder, such as systemic lupus erythematosus (SLE). Generalised allergic drug reactions usually involve dermatological manifestations.

Localised allergic drug reactions are more common, and although these may affect most organ systems, dermatological reactions are by far the most common manifestations of drug allergy; these may take many forms (*Table 31*). The drugs most frequently implicated in allergic skin reactions are listed in *Table 32*, and it is always very important to remember the possibility of undeclared prescribed or self-medication in taking a history from a patient with a dermatological condition (*Table 33*).

Table 29. *Clinical criteria for drug allergy.**

- The observed manifestations do not resemble the pharmacological action of the drug.
- The reactions are generally similar to those which may occur with other allergens.
- An induction period, commonly 7–10 days, is required following initial exposure to the drug.
- The reaction may be reproduced by cross-reacting chemical structures.
- The reaction may be reproduced by minute doses of the drug.
- Blood and/or tissue eosinophilia may be present.
- Discontinuation of the drug results in resolution of the reaction.
- The reaction occurs in a minority of patients receiving the drug.

*Similar principles apply to allergy to any ingested substance, but their assessment may be complicated by chronicity of ingestion.

Table 30. *Differences between non-allergic and allergic drug reactions.*

Difference	Non-allergic	Allergic
Quantities required to provoke reaction	Large	Minute
Cumulative effect	Often necessary	Usually none
Relationship between allergic effect and pharmacological action	Often present	No connection
Same effect reproduced by pharmacologically different chemicals	Rare	Common
Clinical picture	Uniform	Varied

Table 31. *Clinical manifestations of drug allergy in the skin.*

Manifestation	Figure
Erythematous maculopapular eruption (50%)	187–190
Urticaria/angioedema (25%)	24, 48, 191
Contact dermatitis	163, 164, 192
Fixed drug eruption	193
Erythema multiforme/ Stevens–Johnson syndrome	10, 131, 132, 194, 195
Exfoliative dermatitis	196
Photosensitivity	182, 183, 197
Vasculitis	198
Erythema nodosum	129, 130, 199
Toxic epidermal necrolysis	200, 201
Erythematosquamous eruption	202

Table 32. *Drugs frequently implicated in allergic skin reactions.*

- Aspirin
- NSAIDs
- Penicillins
- Sulphonamides
- Antituberculous drugs
- Nitrofurans
- Antimalarials
- Griseofulvin
- Hypnotics
- Anticonvulsants
- Tranquillisers
- Antihypertensives
- Anti-arrhythmics
- Antisera and vaccines
- Organ extracts, e.g. insulin, ACTH
- Heavy metals
- Allopurinol
- Penicillamine
- Antithyroid drugs

Table 33. *Medication often overlooked as a cause of skin reactions.*[*]

- Aspirin and other analgesics
- Nose drops
- Cold 'cures'
- Sedatives
- Laxatives
- Antibiotics
- Tonics
- Contraceptives
- Ointments
- Douches
- Suppositories
- Lozenges
- Dysmenorrhoea treatment

[*] i.e. considered unimportant by the patient. The doctor should specifically ask about each medication.

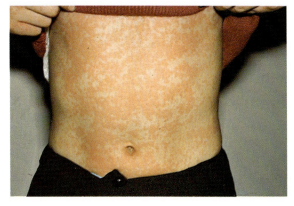

187 Erythematous maculopapular eruption in a patient who had been treated with penicillin. Eruptions of this kind are by far the most common manifestation of allergy to drugs, although similar appearances may undoubtedly also occur through non-allergic mechanisms. In this case, some of the lesions were papules, but drug-induced rashes may also be macular or morbilliform (visible, but not palpable).

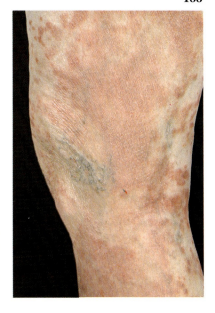

188 Erythematous maculopapular eruption following ampicillin administration. This patient seemed to have a true allergy to drugs containing a penicilloyl group, but similar rashes are very common in patients with infectious mononucleosis, whose symptoms have initially been treated with ampicillin. In that setting, the rash seems to result from a non-allergic interaction between the drug and the disease.

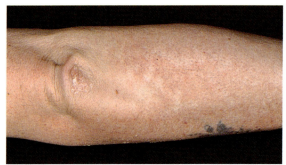 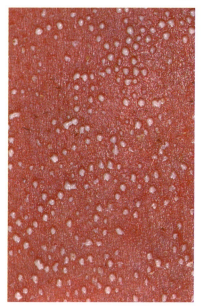

189, 190 A pustular reaction occurred in this patient following the use of iodinated contrast medium during coronary angiography. At a glance, the reaction appears erythematous (**189**), but closer inspection (**190**) reveals the presence of multiple small pustules. Many halogenated compounds are capable of producing this reaction; when produced by iodine, it is also known as 'iododerma'. The reaction was generalised and symmetrical. Its mechanism is unknown, and immunological factors may not be involved.

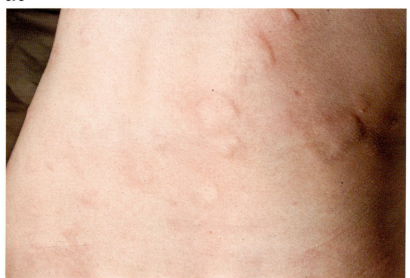

191 Acute urticaria is a common manifestation of drug allergy. The weals disappear without trace – usually after no more than a few hours. Aspirin and related non-steroidal anti-inflammatory drugs, penicillins, and blood products are the most frequent causes of urticarial drug eruptions, but many other drugs may cause similar symptoms. In severe cases, angioedema or a systemic anaphylactic reaction may occur (see **24** and Chapter 4).

192 Contact dermatitis resulting from allergy to ear drops. This woman had a mild otitis externa, which became much more severe after treatment with chloramphenicol ear drops. Contact sensitivity to chloramphenicol is quite common, and a similar reaction may result from the use of drops containing neomycin. Similar reactions may result from the use of eye drops or ointments containing these antibiotics.

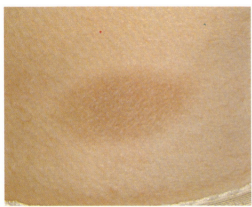

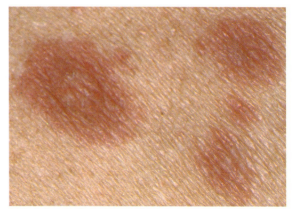

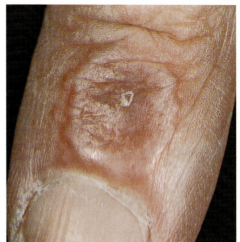

193 A fixed drug eruption, so called because the lesion recurs at the same site after each administration of the causative drug. Fixed drug eruptions are often misdiagnosed, as they are so localised. In this patient the cause was barbiturates, but similar reactions may occur to many other drugs, including various over-the-counter laxative preparations containing phenolphthalein.

194, 195 Erythema multiforme may follow the administration of a range of drugs. In this case the cause was sulphonamide therapy. Note the characteristic target-like lesions (see also **10, 131, 132**). The lesion seen in **195** has blistered in the centre. This is consistent with the diagnosis of erythema multiforme, but blistering does not always occur.

196 Exfoliative dermatitis is a severe complication of drug sensitivity, which may require a period of intensive medical care. If the reaction is generalised, the patient may suffer from a failure of normal temperature regulation, from excessive fluid loss, and from secondary infection. This 25-year-old African man developed generalised exfoliative dermatitis following co-trimoxazole therapy.

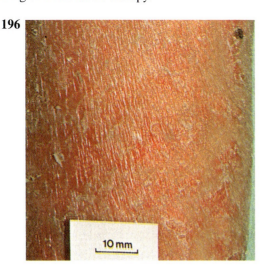

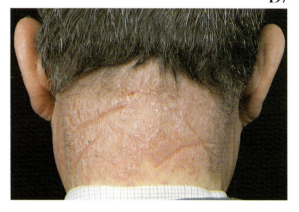

197 A photoallergic drug reaction resulted from doxycycline therapy in this patient. Note how the reaction ceases at the line of his collar. The relationship to light exposure is clear here, but it may not always be so obvious. Not all such reactions are truly allergic in origin – phototoxicity is more common than photoallergy, and airborne contact dermatitis is also limited to exposed areas (see Chapters 7 and 8).

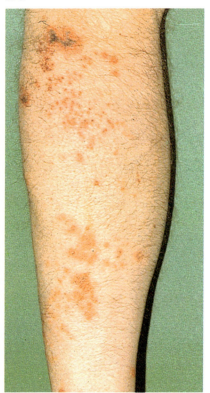 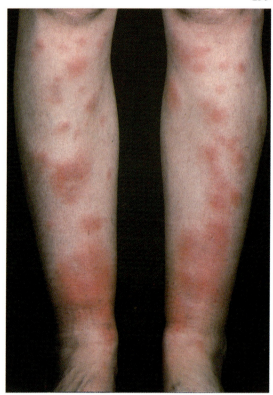

198 Vasculitis must be considered if an eruption is purpuric and palpable. This 51-year-old man developed vasculitis following treatment with penicillin, but similar reactions may be seen in response to a number of other drugs.

199 Erythema nodosum may be induced by oral contraceptives and by sulphonamide therapy. In appearance, it is identical to erythema nodosum resulting from other causes (see **129** and **130**). The deep inflammation of subcutaneous fat and vasculature gives characteristic tender, red nodules on the lower legs and, sometimes, the forearms.

Management of allergy to drugs

When an allergic drug reaction is suspected, the drug should be withdrawn. If the patient is receiving multiple drug therapy for a major disease, this may prove a complex task, but the drugs listed in *Tables 32* and *33* should always be considered as major suspects. The linking of some drugs to particular allergic manifestations may provide important clues to the likely culprit drug – e.g. sulphonamides causing erythema multiforme, or penicillins causing urticaria or angioedema.

Skin prick tests are hazardous in drug allergy, and neither they nor *in vitro* tests can be clearly interpreted in every case. Patch tests also have a very limited role in the diagnosis of drug allergy: they may be useful where topical therapy is suspected of causing an eczematous eruption, but they have no other uses.

The manifestations of drug allergy may require treatment in their own right:

- Angioedema with laryngeal involvement or anaphylaxis may need immediate treatment with injected adrenaline and hydrocortisone.
- Generalised life-threatening eruptions, such as the Stevens–Johnson syndrome or exfoliative dermatitis, may need urgent intensive care, with fluid replacement and the prevention or treatment of secondary infection. Steroid treatment probably has a role in some conditions, but has been shown not to be beneficial in the Stevens–Johnson syndrome.
- Patients with pruritic eruptions may be helped by oral antihistamine treatment, and by local treatment with simple calamine lotion or 2% menthol in calamine cream.

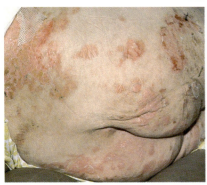 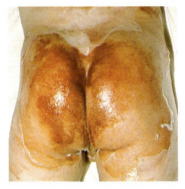 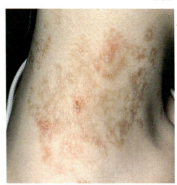

200 Toxic epidermal necrolysis (also known as the 'scalded skin syndrome') is a condition in which large areas of skin become bright red, then slough at the dermoepidermal border. It can be clinically similar to the staphylococcal scalded skin syndrome, which usually occurs in infants and is induced by a staphylococcal toxin (though the split in that syndrome is usually high in the epidermis). Toxic epidermal necrolysis is often an extreme manifestation of the Stevens–Johnson syndrome. It is most commonly caused by sulphonamide therapy, as in this elderly woman, but other drugs are sometimes implicated. When large areas of the skin are affected, it is a potentially life-threatening condition, with a high risk of complications in survivors, including corneal scarring.

201 Toxic epidermal necrolysis. In this young boy the condition followed phenytoin therapy. Loss of such large areas of skin requires intensive nursing therapy. The condition requires urgent specialist treatment as it can be fatal, and secondary infection of the exposed areas is a major problem.

202 An erythematosquamous eruption is the most common manifestation of allergy to gold therapy. This patient with rheumatoid arthritis developed a widespread eruption, which persisted after withdrawal of therapy.

Once true allergy to a drug has been established, further administration of that drug or other cross-reacting drugs should be avoided unless there is no alternative. It is sometimes possible to desensitise a patient to a drug by giving repeated doses under close supervision in hospital, but the effect of this manoeuvre is short-lived unless drug administration is subsequently continuous, so it is only applicable where long-term therapy with the culprit drug is essential.

Food Allergy and the Skin

Adverse reactions to food can be categorised in the same way as adverse reactions to drugs:

- Non-allergic causes.
- Idiosyncratic causes.
- Allergic causes.

Non-allergic adverse reactions include a wide range of metabolic disorders and the consequences of poisoning by a wide range of substances.

Allergy and non-immunological idiosyncrasy to food may be grouped together as 'food intolerance'. Either may provoke dermatological abnormalities, but, as discussed above, their role is not so obvious or so widely agreed as that of drugs. At present, food intolerance is known to have a role in a limited number of conditions, including:

- Urticaria/angioedema.
- Atopic eczema.
- Dermatitis herpetiformis.

Food intolerance in urticaria and angioedema

The most clear-cut example of a food-induced dermatological disorder is the urticaria and angioedema which may follow the ingestion of specific foods in susceptible individuals (203). Many cases clearly result from isolated foods (such as shellfish, strawberries, and peanuts), and some patients may experience similar symptoms after the ingestion of foods which contain natural salicylates (in which case they will usually react similarly to aspirin), azo-dyes (such as tartrazine) which are used as food colourings, or benzoic acid and its derivatives which are used as food preservatives.

Within minutes of the ingestion of the food, the affected individual experiences itching and swelling of the lips and mouth. In severe cases this may be followed by a widespread – but usually short-lived – urticarial reaction, by vomiting (a manifestation of a lower gastrointestinal involvement), or, most seriously, by pharyngeal or laryngeal oedema with respiratory obstruction and even anaphylaxis. The reaction is rarely fatal; at the other end of the spectrum, it may be no more than a trivial irritant to the patients.

These reactions have the characteristics of an immediate IgE-mediated allergic response, and in some cases this is clearly the mechanism. Specific, positive skin prick reactions may be found – e.g. to peanuts – and a positive radioallergosorbent test (RAST) may provide confirmation of immunological reactivity. In many cases, however, substances from the offending foods seem to trigger direct mediator release in a susceptible individual; this produces identical symptoms and signs by a non-immunological mechanism.

In an individual patient the mechanism of the response is often unclear, and investigations are commonly inconclusive (*Table 34*); but fortunately

Table 34. *Investigations in suspected food intolerance.*

- There are no reliable laboratory tests for food allergy or idiosyncrasy.
- Skin prick testing with a few food extracts (such as egg, fish, nuts, and yeast) gives results which correlate well with clinical symptoms, but positive results tend to persist even when clinical sensitivity has been lost.
- Skin prick testing is difficult to interpret where the patient has dermographism or widespread eczema.
- Serum IgE may be raised in an allergic response, but this does not demonstrate that the responsible antigen entered via the gut.
- Radioallergosorbent tests for specific IgE antibodies may sometimes demonstrate raised circulating antibody levels to specific foods, but for most of the food extracts used the correlation with symptoms is poor.
- Skin and small-bowel biopsy confirm the diagnosis of dermatitis herpetiformis.
- 'Fringe' techniques (such as sublingual or cytotoxic food tests, hair analysis, etc.) are widely advertised but valueless.
- A diagnostic exclusion diet, followed by appropriate food challenge, is the mainstay of investigation.

this has little practical significance, as the management of these patients is similar whether or not a true allergic mechanism lies behind the symptoms. Where the provoking food is obvious, it should be avoided if possible. Where it is not, the possibility of sensitivity to salicylates or tartrazine in food should be considered, and a trial period on an exclusion diet may prove diagnostic (see below). Urticaria and angioedema, which are not clearly related to food intake, rarely respond to exclusion diets, however, and food intolerance is probably only a rare cause of chronic urticaria and angioedema.

The general management of established food

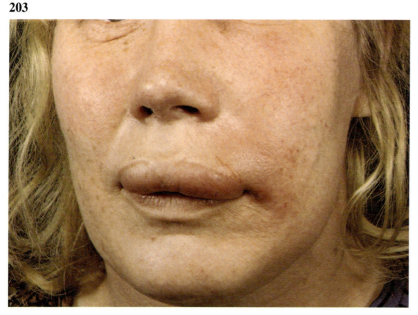

203 Angioedema may follow the ingestion of specific food by susceptible individuals. This patient had a relatively mild reaction, with swelling of the lip, but in severe cases the face may be grossly swollen, and pharyngeal and laryngeal oedema may lead to respiratory obstruction. Often a food is clearly responsible, but, as a recent series of case reports on allergy to peanuts has shown, it is not always easy to avoid types of food which are widely used in catering or pre-packed foods. Food allergy of this type can occasionally prove fatal.

Table 35. *The management of food intolerance in the skin.*

- Isolated reactions to foods which can be avoided (strawberries, shellfish, etc.) are best managed by simple avoidance.
- Multiple intolerance (especially when it involves intolerance to cow's milk, eggs, yeast, etc.) can be managed by a more rigorous therapeutic exclusion diet, but this must be carefully planned and monitored to ensure nutritional adequacy, and compliance with the diet is often a problem.
- Desensitisation therapy using injections, or by oral or nasal administration, has been advocated by some, but no scientific or controlled clinical studies support the use of these techniques.
- There is no preventive drug treatment for food allergy or idiosyncracy, though oral sodium cromoglycate may have occasional value as an adjunct to diet in multiple food allergy. The appropriate dose of the drug is not known, and probably varies widely from one patient to another.
- Antihistamines and, occasionally, corticosteroids may be needed for symptomatic treatment.
- Adverse responses to food may change with time, and problem foods should be reintroduced on a trial basis at intervals.
- Dermatitis herpetiformis is a special case, requiring treatment with dapsone and a gluten-free diet.
- For eczema and urticaria, symptomatic treatment is often necessary and effective; and it may be preferable to a prolonged exclusion diet and/or a useful additional part of the therapy.

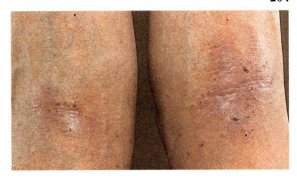

204 Infantile atopic eczema. Note the excoriated, lichenified dermatitis in the knee flexures. At this stage, some children show an improvement if cow's milk, egg, or other substances are eliminated from their diet. However, atopic eczema is rarely – if ever – due to food allergy alone.

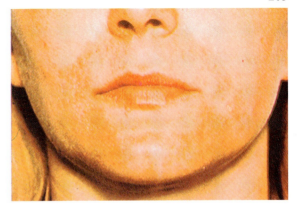

205 Eczema resulting from orange drink. This adult patient suspected that her perioral dermatitis might be caused by ingested substances, and its distribution was different from typical perioral eczema. An exclusion diet showed the cause to be the food colouring azo-dyes tartrazine (E102) and sunset yellow (E110), and not orange juice itself (but note that citrus fruits are among the commoner causes of food-related symptoms).

intolerance is summarised in *Table 35*. Patients with acute urticaria or angioedema may respond to antihistamine treatment, and this may be of value prophylactically, where exposure to provoking foods is difficult to avoid – during international travel, for example. Corticosteriod therapy or even injected adrenaline may be necessary for severe or life-threatening angioedema.

Food intolerance in atopic eczema

Eczema is a complex disease, involving Type I and Type IV immune responses and other processes (see Chapter 10). It is likely that it can be influenced by many factors, and that dietary factors may play a role. This may be a relatively minor role in many patients, but occasionally – especially in infants – allergy or idiosyncrasy to foods may play a more major role in the genesis of eczema, or in determining its severity (**204, 205**).

Some children with generalised infantile atopic eczema show an improvement if cow's milk, egg, or – sometimes – other substances are eliminated from their diet. In some of these patients there is evidence from skin prick testing or RAST studies to suggest a specific Type I IgE-mediated hypersensitivity to egg or cow's milk protein. Skin prick testing is, however, an unreliable technique in eczematous patients, because false-positive results are common; and the levels of IgE found by RAST do not show a good correlation with disease activity. It is doubtful whether allergy to foods is the sole cause of eczema in these patients, but it may influence its severity.

In older children and adults, similar abnormalities in skin prick test results and RASTs may be found, but formal studies suggest that dietary modification has little or no part to play in management. Individual patients (often encouraged by 'fringe' practitioners) occasionally report dramatic improvements, but these are very difficult to assess against the background of a condition of naturally variable severity.

It is impracticable to assess the effect of diagnostic exclusion diets in all patients with atopic eczema. Those with mild disease should usually be treated symptomatically, and an exclusion diet should only be used if there is a strong clinical suspicion (by the patient, the patient's parents, or the physician) that specific foods may play a role. This suspicion will usually occur more often in infantile eczema than in eczema later in life. In older patients there may be a case for a trial of an exclusion diet if the eczema is difficult to control, and if the patient is keen to investigate all possible approaches to treatment – but the chance of success is very low, and this should be clearly explained to the patient before embarking on the difficulties associated with such a diet (see below).

Dermatitis herpetifomis

The blistering skin disease dermatitis herpetiformis is always associated with a gluten-sensitive enteropathy resembling coeliac disease, and both conditions respond to the complete exclusion of gluten from the diet – though the response of the skin eruption may be slow, in which case the addition of dapsone therapy may speed up its resolution.

There is clear evidence of multiple immunological abnormalities in both coeliac disease and dermatitis herpetiformis, including the frequent presence of circulating antigliadin and antireticulin antibodies. It seems likely that immunological abnormalities are the primary cause of the disease, but this is not fully proven; it is possible that gluten induces initial damage by non-immunological means, and that the immunological changes are a secondary phenomenon.

Table 36. *Diagnostic exclusion diets appropriate for possibly food-related symptoms in the skin.*

Condition	Diagnostic Diet
Urticaria or angioedema	Azo-dye, benzoic acid, and salicylate free*
Eczema	Cow's milk and egg free[a]
Dermatitis herpetiformis	Gluten free†

* A full exclusion diet should be tried if a more specific diet is unsuccessful.
† Dermatitis herpetiformis is usually diagnosed on skin biopsy with immunofluorescence, but dietary treatment is usually indicated.

Diagnostic and therapeutic exclusion diets in eczema and urticaria/angioedema

A 'full exclusion diet' is very restricted. The precise recommended content varies from one centre to another, but the common aim is to exclude all foods which could provoke symptoms. Many patients find it difficult to adhere to a full exclusion diet, and for skin conditions it is usually possible to use a less restricted diet in the first instance, following this with a period on a full exclusion diet if necessary (*Table 36*).

The patient should keep a detailed food diary throughout the exclusion period. If the symptoms do not remit during 2–3 weeks on this diet, food or food additives are an unlikely cause of symptoms. Further investigation and/or symptomatic treatments are then indicated.

If the symptoms remit when on the diet, the patients should reintroduce all the excluded foods one at a time, at intervals of 2–7 days over the next few months, while continuing on a gradually expanding exclusion diet throughout this period (composed of the original diet together with additional foods as and when they are shown not to cause symptoms). Foods should be introduced in order of importance in a normal diet – e.g. tap water first, followed by potatoes, cow's milk, yeast, etc. However, if the patient suspects individual excluded foods of causing symptoms, these should be reintroduced early in the second phase, as a response to their reintroduction may make further investigation unnecessary.

The role of individual foods can be confirmed by the 'blind' administration of freeze-dried food in unmarked capsules, so that the patient is unaware of the nature of the food under test. This technique has the limitation of small volume, which should not affect true allergic responses, but may prevent adverse responses of other kinds. It also prevents the food from coming into contact with the lips, mouth, and oesophagus, and may not reproduce symptoms related to these organs. In practice, the technique is usually reserved for formal studies; it has a limited role in routine investigation.

10 Eczema and Dermatitis

The terms 'eczema' and 'dermatitis' are best regarded as synonyms. They refer to a type of skin inflammation with characteristic clinical and histological features. The clinical manifestations include erythema, vesiculation, weeping, and scaling, and the histological features are shown in **206**. They are similar in exogenous and endogenous dermatitis.

The classification of both eczema and dermatitis is difficult. The disorders may be acute, subacute, or chronic. The most commonly used subdivision is:

- Exogenous (or contact) eczema/dermatitis.
- Endogenous (or constitutional) eczema/dermatitis

A further convenient subdivision is shown in Table 37.

Dermatitis is a common cause of dermatological symptoms and a frequent reason for referral to the dermatology clinic. Although the classic presentations of atopic eczema and contact dermatitis are often easily diagnosed, it is important to remember both a range of treatable conditions which may be confused with these conditions (*Table 38*) and a number of rare conditions which may produce eczema-like changes in the skin (*Table 39*).

Table 37. *A classification of dermatitis or eczema.*

Exogenous (contact)	Irritant
	Allergic
	Photodermatitis
Endogenous (constitutional)	Atopic
	Seborrhoeic
	Nummular (discoid)
	Pompholyx (dyshidrotic)
	Varicose/gravitational/stasis
Unclassified	Asteatotic
	Neurodermatitis/lichen simplex chronicus
	Nodular prurigo
	Lichen striatus

Table 38. *Conditions often confused with eczema.*

Fungal infections
Psoriasis
Scabies
Pityriasis rosea
Secondary syphilis
Drug reactions in photodermatitis
Erysipelas
Icthyosis
Acrodermatitis enteropathica
Histiocytosis X
X-linked agamma-globulinaemia

Table 39. *Some unusual causes of eczematous skin changes.*

Phenylketonuria
Wiskoff–Aldrich syndrome
Anhidrotic epidermal dysplasia
Pellagra
Malabsorption (essential fatty acids)

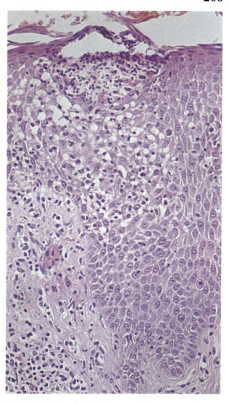

206 Histopathology of eczematous reaction. This is a high-power view of the epidermis and papillary dermis in atopic eczema. There is epidermal thinning (acanthosis) and oedema (spongiosis), with a moderately heavy mononuclear cell infiltrate in the superficial dermis and epidermis (exocytosis). These features are seen in both exogenous and endogenous eczema; they are not specific to one subtype. The subcorneal pustule represents secondary impetiginisation.

Exogenous Dermatitis

Exogenous or contact dermatitis is relatively simple to define as an eczematous eruption produced by external agents. The reaction may be acute or chronic, and it may be produced by Type IV allergic mechanisms, directly by irritants, or by photosensitive reactions (allergic or non-allergic). Contact irritant dermatitis is much commoner than contact allergic dermatitis, accounting for around 80% of cases of contact dermatitis.

In differential diagnosis, contact dermatitis is likely if:

- There is obvious contact with known irritants or allergens.
- The eruption clears when the patient goes on holiday or at weekends (in occupational dermatitis).
- The eczema is asymmetrical (**207**), or has a linear or rectilinear configuration.

The eruption often involves the eyelids, external ear canals, hands, feet, and perianal skin.

Contact dermatitis is reviewed in detail in Chapter 7, and photodermatitis – another form of exogenous dermatitis – is reviewed in Chapter 8.

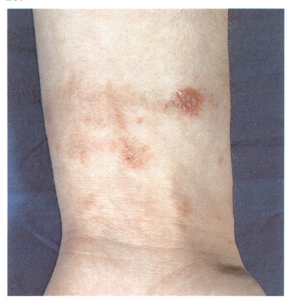

207 Contact allergic dermatitis to nickel. This young woman had developed a Type IV Gell and Coombs hypersensitivity reaction to nickel in the buckle of her watch strap. This has resulted in an asymmetrical exogenous contact allergic dermatitis (see also Chapter 7).

Endogenous Dermatitis

Atopic eczema

Since its aetiology and pathogenesis are unknown, atopic eczema is difficult to define. It is an endogenous dermatitis affecting young children predominantly, but not exclusively. It is characterised by itchy epidermal lesions and runs a chronic and relapsing course. Most patients have raised circulating IgE levels, there is a genetic predisposition to the disease, and it is commonly associated with a personal or family history of atopic disease, such as asthma and hay fever. Multiple positive immediate skin prick tests to commonly tested allergens (see Chapter 3) are often present. Defective cell-mediated immunity and fluctuation in the *in vivo* expression of cell-mediated immunity are also reported.

Type I allergic mechanisms may play a role in the early stages of the disease, but – despite the continuing association with other Type I reactions – it seems likely that many later features of the disease are manifestations of Type IV delayed hypersensitivity or other abnormalities (see also Chapters 4 and 7). Evidence is accumulating that atopic eczema in children may represent a cutaneous manifestation of allergy to a wide variety of environmental allergens, including some in food and possibly the house dust mite.

Atopic eczema affects about 5% of the population, and it usually begins before the age of 6 months. The distribution and character of the lesions vary with age, and the typical appearances are discussed and illustrated in Chapter 4 (**61–65**). The changes in distribution are illustrated diagramatically in **208**, and a range of typical appearances is shown in **209–213** (see also Chapters 1 and 4). Atopic eczema remits spontaneously in 65% of affected children before they are 10 years of age, but most patients have generally dry skin throughout life. A rare complication in patients with chronic atopic eczema is the development of cataracts.

Other skin conditions which may be associated with atopic eczema or the atopic state include keratosis pilaris (**214**), pityriasis alba (**215**), and juvenile plantar dermatosis (**216**).

Chronic atopic eczema may be complicated by a range of secondary infections. Typical examples are shown in **209** and **217–221**.

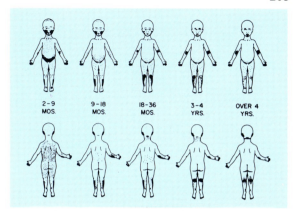

208 The distribution of atopic eczema varies with age. Infantile eczema predominantly involves the cheeks and trunk, whereas from childhood onwards, the eczema is mainly confined to the flexures (see also Chapter 4).

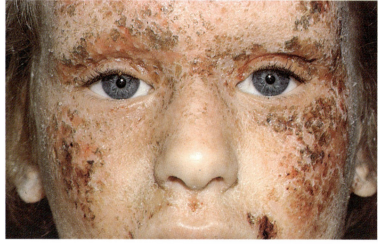

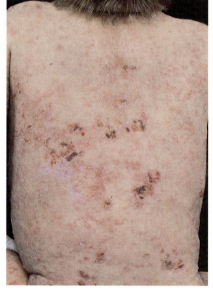

209 Acute atopic eczema with impetiginisation. Involvement of the face is common in infancy. In this patient, the eczema was complicated by secondary infection with *Staphylococcus aureus*. Treatment required both topical corticosteroids and systemic antibiotics.

210 Atopic eczema affecting the trunk. This is usually patchy and crusted without particular involvement of the flexures. This young girl has widespread erythema and severe pruritus. She required admission for intensive in-patient therapy.

211 Reverse pattern atopic eczema. In Afro-Caribbeans, atopic eczema tends to be more lichenified and papular, and it sometimes affects the extensor surfaces, rather than the flexures.

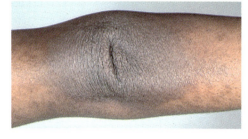

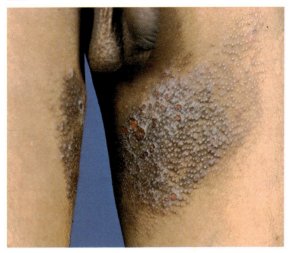

212 Lichenified atopic eczema. Prolonged scratching and rubbing can lead to severe hyperpigmentation and lichenification. If localised, the condition is known as lichen simplex.

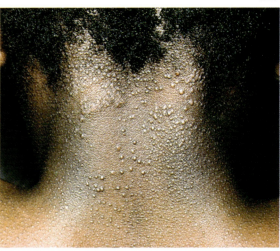

213 Papular atopic eczema. This young girl demonstrates the papular type of lichenification, which has occurred over the nape of her neck following prolonged scratching and rubbing of her atopic eczema.

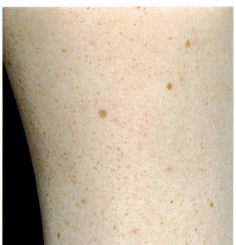

214 Keratosis pilaris. This condition is a relatively common autosomal dominant disorder due to hyperkeratosis of the hair follicles, which become filled with horny plugs. The changes begin in childhood and improve with age. They are usually confined to the outer aspects of the arms and thighs and rarely involve the face. Association with atopy is recognised.

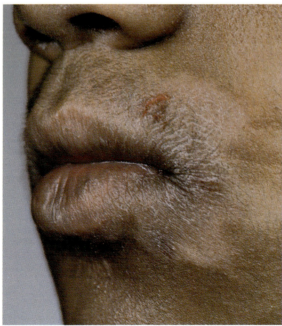

215 Pityriasis alba. This is characterised by hypopigmented scaly patches in the perioral region, on the cheeks, and sometimes on the proximal limbs. It is found in otherwise normal patients and in those with atopic eczema. It inevitably resolves with age.

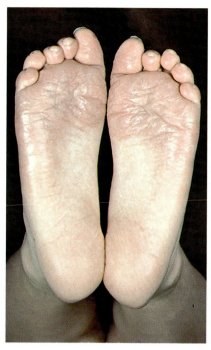

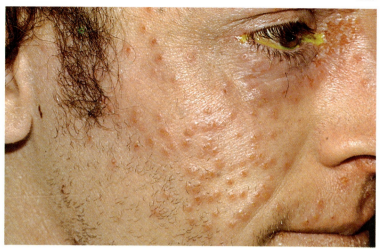

216 Juvenile plantar dermatosis. Some feel this condition is a manifestation of atopy. The skin of the weight-bearing areas of the feet becomes dry and shiny, with deep painful fissures. Trainer shoes, which are popular among children, often cause excessive sweating and may be the true culprit.

217 Eczema herpeticum (Kaposi's varicelliform eruption). This man with atopic eczema developed a cold sore, which spread to cause a severe vesicular eruption on the face. It is important to refer such patients to the ophthalmologist, as involvement of the cornea can lead to dendritic ulceration, scarring, and permanent visual impairment.

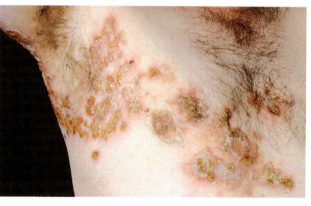

218 Herpes zoster in eczema. This young man with atopic eczema developed shingles of the T4 dermatome. The eruption became secondarily infected with *Staphylococcus aureus*, i.e. impetiginised. Patients with atopic eczema are more susceptible to skin infections.

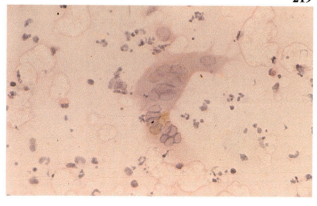

219 Herpes infection. A Tzanck test is useful in confirming a herpetic infection, whether simplex or zoster. This is performed by removing the roof of a fresh vesicle, scraping the base, and examining the cells microscopically. The cells here are multinucleated, which confirms a viral infection.

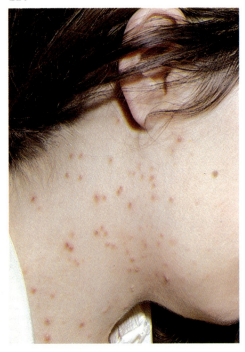

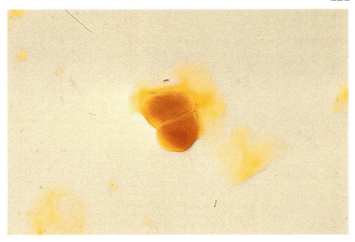

220 Molluscum contagiosum. This young girl with atopic eczema developed numerous umbilicated erythematous papules over the neck. Some discharged pus-like material. Staining revealed molluscum bodies. Molluscum contagiosum is due to a pox virus which usually affects young children who develop a few lesions. However, in atopic subjects the infection can be widespread.

221 Molluscum bodies. Light microscopy on stained cheesy material expressed from a lesion shows that many of the keratinocytes contain oval, darkly staining aggregations of pox virus particles, which confirms the diagnosis of molluscum contagiosum.

Seborrhoeic eczema

Seborrhoeic eczema is usually confined to areas richly populated with sebaceous glands. Perifollicular, erythematous pink or yellow lesions which develop into macular patches appear on the scalp and face (**222**), and in the retroauricular, pre-sternal, interscapular, and intertriginous areas. Typical eczematous changes are seen only occasionally. Increased sebum production and hyperhidrosis provide a base for microbial action and inflammatory changes. In infants, seborrhoeic eczema may present as cradle cap but clears rapidly; in adults it may be chronic.

An overgrowth of *Pityrosporum*, commonly found in this condition, is thought by many clinicians to be important in the pathogenesis of seborrhoeic dermatitis.

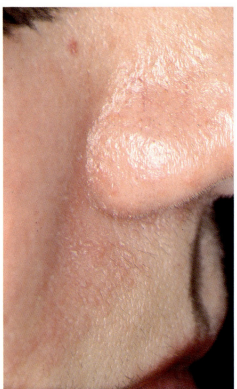

222 Seborrhoeic eczema. This young lady complained of an erythematous, scaly eruption of her face affecting her nasolabial folds. It appeared to improve in sunshine and responded to topical antifungal agents together with mild corticosteroids. Other areas affected include the scalp, chest, and sometimes the groin.

Nummular or discoid eczema

Nummular (discoid) eczema is characterised by pruritic, coin-like, oozing patches, frequently located on the extensor surfaces, and is commonest in middle-aged men (223). In patients with an atopic history, it may be considered to be an exudative form of neurodermatitis – in contrast to the dry form, which is called lichen simplex.

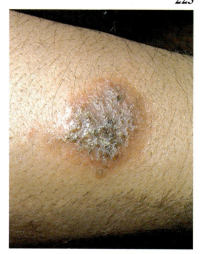

223 Nummular discoid eczema. This young man complained of a pruritic erythematous scaly patch on the outer aspect of his forearm. Repeated skin scrapings failed to show any infection; in particular, no fungal elements were found. Once the area had been occluded and treated with topical corticosteroids, there was a marked improvement. The lower legs are also a common site for nummular eczema.

Pompholyx

Pompholyx can be unpleasant. Recurrent vesicles or bullae affect the palms, fingers, and/or soles of adults (**167, 224, 225**). It is characterised by remissions and relapses, which are sometimes provoked by heat, emotional stress, or an active fungal infection of the feet. There have been reports that the ingestion of small amounts of nickel in susceptible patients may trigger an attack.

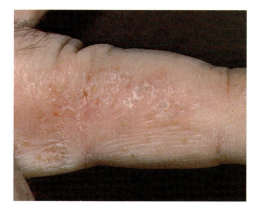

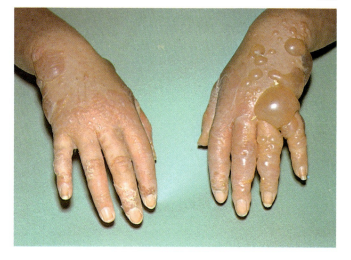

224 Pompholyx. This young man developed pruritic vesicles on the lateral aspects of many of his fingers, especially when he was under stress. The eruption resolved with regular use of emollients and topical corticosteroids – sometimes used under occlusion.

225 Pompholyx. In this middle-aged lady the vesicles had become more extensive, coalescing to form large, painful fluid-filled bullae. She also had involvement of the plantar aspect of her feet. This degree of endogenous eczema required urgent admission, decompression of the blisters, and topical corticosteroid treatment, often under occlusive bandages. Secondary infection usually occurs and requires treatment with systemic antibiotics.

Varicose eczema

Varicose eczema presents as a chronic condition, affecting the lower legs of middle-aged and elderly patients (**226**). It is often accompanied by venous insufficiency, with obvious varicose veins, oedema, haemosiderin deposition, and lipodermatosclerosis. The venous insufficiency may lead to ulcer formation. Topical medicaments used in venous ulceration can aggravate the condition by causing contact allergic dermatitis in addition to the underlying stasis eczema.

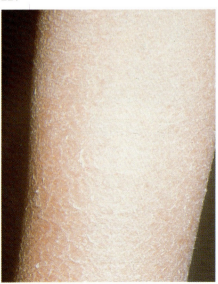

226 Varicose eczema. This middle-aged man has severe venous insufficiency, demonstrated by haemosiderin deposition in the skin of his lower legs. In the past he had also developed a venous ulcer and he is troubled by prutitus due to stasis eczema. This endogenous eczema can be complicated by contact allergic dermatitis to topical medicaments, such as neomycin. If this is suspected, patch testing should be carried out.

Unclassified Dermatitis

Asteatotic eczema

Asteatotic eczema is a common dermatosis which occurs on the legs of elderly patients, but is often unrecognised. Against a background of dry skin, a network of fine red superficial fissures appears, causing a 'crazy paving' appearance (**227**).

227 Asteatotic eczema (eczema crequale). This is a common form of endogenous eczema affecting the elderly. The characteristic fissuring of the skin gives a 'crazy paving' appearance. Often it is well-controlled by avoidance of irritants and the regular use of topical emollients.

Neurodermatitis

Neurodermatitis, or lichen simplex chronicus, usually presents with a single, fixed, lichenified plaque, which is perpetuated by repeated rubbing or scratching, either as a habit or as a response to stress (**212, 228**). Favourite sites are the nape of neck in women, the legs in men, and the anogenital area in both sexes. Lesions tend to be chronic.

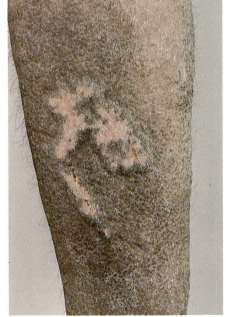

228 Lichen simplex chronicus. This Asian lady developed a large lichenified plaque of eczema on the leg due to intense scratching. The end result was post-inflammatory hypopigmentation. Treatment, as with nodular prurigo, is often difficult, requiring occlusive therapy, usually with strong topical corticosteroids, antihistamines, and regular use of emollients.

Nodular prurigo

Nodular prurigo, in many respects, resembles lichen simplex, often affecting middle-aged women. Individual lesions are hard symmetrical nodules, often on the proximal parts of the limbs (**229**). The itching is severe and the course is chronic. The cause is unknown, although emotional stress seems contributory in some cases, and iron deficiency may play a role in others.

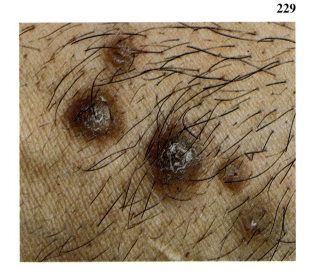

229 Nodular prurigo. This condition usually affects middle-aged and elderly females who present with pruritic nodules on the legs and arms. A few cases may have an underlying iron-deficiency, but the majority are a form of neurodermatitis.

Lichen striatus

Lichen striatus is an unusual self-limiting inflammatory linear dermatitis of unknown origin (**230**). Over 50% of cases occur in children, particularly in females. It can be asymptomatic. Spontaneous cure can be expected within 3–6 months in most cases. Temporary hyperpigmentation may result in coloured skin.

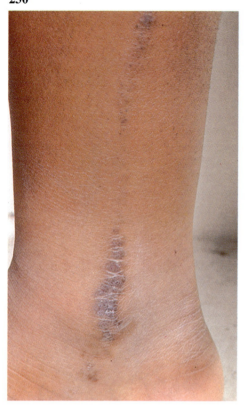

230 Lichen striatus. This condition often presents in children as a linear form of eczema, particularly in females. It is not necessarily pruritic. It may produce hyperpigmentation, as in this young Asian girl. The condition is usually self-limiting. Its aetiology is unknown.

11 Management of Allergic Skin Disorders

The management of many individual disorders has been outlined in previous chapters. In this chapter we review the principles of management for each group of disorders and examine in more detail the management of eczema/dermatitis.

Type I Reactions

In urticaria, the ideal approach is to find the cause and eliminate it. Mast cell degranulators, such as aspirin and non-steroidal anti-inflammatory drugs, and opiates, such as codeine and morphine, should be avoided. Some tips for individual subtypes are given in *Table 11*. In general, antihistamines are the mainstay of symptomatic treatment. Newer, non-sedating antihistamines are particularly useful, because if the eruption is not controlled with the initial dosage, the dose can often be increased without side-effects. H_2-blocking antihistamines may add a slight benefit if used together with an H_1-antagonist. Sympathomimetic agents and systemic corticosteroids should only be used in an emergency. In some cases an elimination diet may prove useful. For further details, see Chapters 4 and 9.

Type II Reactions

Bullous dermatoses

The severe group of bullous dermatoses, including pemphigus, pemphigoid, and herpes gestationis, often requires high-dose systemic corticosteroids and/or other immunosuppressive drugs. Dermatitis herpetiformis responds slowly to a gluten-free diet, but many patients prefer to take dapsone or sulphapyridine. For further details, see Chapter 5.

Non-bullous dermatoses

Similarly, the non-bullous dermatoses require immunosuppressive treatment, often including high-dose systemic corticosteroids. Local dermatoses, like discoid lupus erythematosus (LE), often respond to topical corticosteroids, but systemic involvement – as in SLE – requires systemic corticosteroids and other imunosuppressive agents, like azathioprine and cyclophosphamide. Antimalarial drugs may also be useful in LE. Sun avoidance and sunscreens are also essential. See Chapter 5 for further details of the management of other Type II disorders.

Type III Reactions

The common cause of Type III reactions is the formation of immune complexes and damage to blood vessels of varying size. Provoking antigens include drugs, autoantigens, and infectious agents, such as bacteria and viruses. The treatment of choice is to identify the cause and eliminate it. If the cause is unknown, bed rest, dapsone, and colchicine may be helpful. Vasculitis affecting the internal organs usually requires immunosuppressive treatment with systemic corticosteroids, or sometimes cyclophosphamide. Cyclosporin A has proved useful in pyoderma gangrenosum. For further details, see Chapter 6.

Type IV Reactions

Management of eczema/dermatitis

The principles of management in dermatitis are similar, whether the diagnosis is atopic eczema or contact dermatitis (*Table 40*). Allergen or irritant avoidance is particularly important in contact dermatitis, and where there is hand involvement (**231**).

Most eczema responds best to topical corticosteroids in an ointment base, and chronic eczema can often be helped by the addition of zinc cream. Depending on the degree of involvement, care must be taken when prescribing excessive corticosteroids. Even for adults, the clinician should be reluctant to prescribe more than 200 g of mildly potent, 50 g of moderately potent, and 30 g of potent topical corticosteroids per week. The amounts of topical corticosteroid needed to cover different body

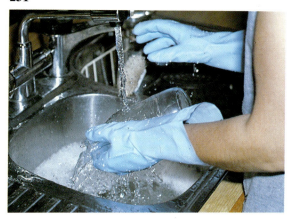

231 Avoidance of irritants in dermatitis of the hand. Whether endogenous or exogenous, involvement of the hands in dermatitis is particularly difficult to treat. The skin should be protected from irritants, such as detergents, and from excessive washing. Rubber gloves (or plastic gloves if the patient is sensitive to rubber) should be worn – ideally with separate, washable cotton linings.

Table 40. *The management of eczema/dermatitis. The principles of management are similar, whatever the cause.*

Patient education
Allergen/irritant avoidance
    Foods/house dust mite in selected patients with atopic eczema
    Allergens/irritants/photosensitisers in contact dermatitis
Topical treatment
Wet dressings
Emollients
    Bath oils
    Ointments
    Creams
    Urea-containing compounds
Corticosteroids
    Ointments/creams
    Weak/moderate/potent/very potent
Tar/ichthammol/zinc

Other treatment (selected cases)
Antimicrobials for secondary infection
    Topical antiseptic
    Topical antibiotic
    Systemic antibiotic
PUVA (psoralens and ultraviolet A)
Oral antihistamines

areas in different age groups are summarised in *Table 41*. It is important to avoid the local (**232**) and systemic side-effects associated with excessive corticosteroid usage. In general, topical corticosteroids should be used intensively for short periods of time, and chronic usage should be avoided whenever possible. Occlusive dressings (**233**) may help to achieve the maximum short-term benefit from topical corticosteroid use.

In the long-term, patients with dermatitis of any cause should avoid soap and use lubricants liberally (**234**). Emollients in the form of emulsifying ointments and aqueous cream are essential. Stabilised urea preparations may be helpful. In chronic cases, particularly of atopic eczema, oral antihistamines may relieve pruritus. Aggravating factors, such as woollen clothes or heat, should always be avoided. Psoralens plus ultraviolet A light (PUVA) therapy has a role in some resistant patients (**235**).

Acute weeping eczema is treated by soaking in a 1:10,000 solution of potassium permanganate, or by other bland treatments. These may be applied as wet dressings (**236**). Impregnated bandages may also be useful, especially as the eczema enters the 'dry' stage (**237**).

Table 41. *Topical corticosteroid therapy (g/week).* *

Age	Whole Body	Both Arms and Legs	Trunk
6 months	35	20	15
1 year	45	25	15
4 years	60	35	20
8 years	90	50	35
12 years	120	65	45
16 years	155	85	55
Adult	170	90	60

*It is important to prescribe an appropriate quantity of corticosteroid for application to the area of skin to be treated. This table gives an indication of the amount required for a twice daily application over 1 week. The total amount required depends on the age of the patient and the area of skin involvement. Although the table specifies the quantity required to treat a given area of skin, it does not imply that the application of potent corticosteroid in this dosage is safe. The choice of strength of corticosteroid must depend on the patient's clinical condition, the duration of therapy, and the site which is involved.

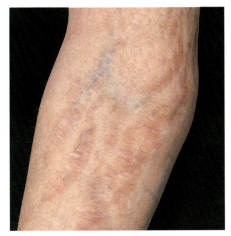

232 Corticosteroid-induced striae. These permanent stretch marks in a patient with atopic eczema were caused by over-use of potent topical corticosteroid therapy. It is essential to avoid the inappropriate and/or excessive use of corticosteroids in such treatment for all dermatological conditions. Additional complications of excessive corticosteroid therapy include delayed healing of wounds, masking of fungal and bacterial infections, and exacerbation of pustular acne.

233 Polythene occlusion. This technique is useful in moderate and severe eczema/dermatitis of any cause. Topical corticosteroid therapy is applied to the treated area, and the area is then occluded with polythene or self-adherent food wrap. This simple technique achieves four major objectives:

- It enhances the penetration of the corticosteroid treatment.
- It prevents the loss of the applied ointment or cream.
- It prevents the patient from scratching or interfering with the healing process.
- It retains the lubrication of the treated area.

This is a valuable technique in the short term, but the enhanced corticosteroid effect carries hazards if the technique is used continually.

235 Localised PUVA therapy. In severe, chronic eczema of the hands and feet, physical modes of treatment may occasionally be helpful. The topical application of a psoralen followed by exposure to ultraviolet A light may give the patient symptomatic relief for several months, but the effects are not permanent. PUVA therapy has more or less replaced the superficial X-ray therapy, which was previously used in selected patients with resistant eczema and has a similar effect.

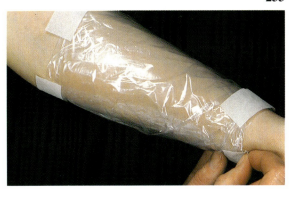

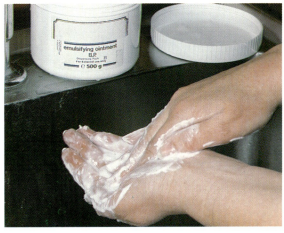

234 Soap substitutes are useful in all types of eczema. They include emulsifying ointment and aqueous cream, and – especially in patients with eczema of the hand – they should always be used in preference to any form of soap or detergent. Many commercial emollients are available, and most can be used on all parts of the body and in bath water.

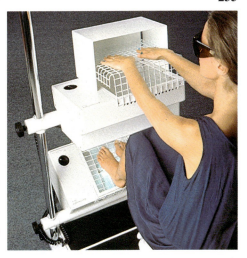

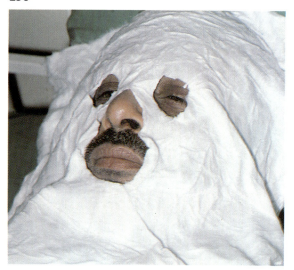

236 Wet wrap therapy. This old-fashioned, but simple, technique is very effective in re-hydrating the skin, and it may be valuable in severe, dry, flaking eczema/dermatitis. The technique also provides considerable symptomatic relief, especially where pruritus is a major problem. If a large part of the body is to be treated in this way, care should be taken to avoid inducing hypothermia as a result of evaporation from the wrap.

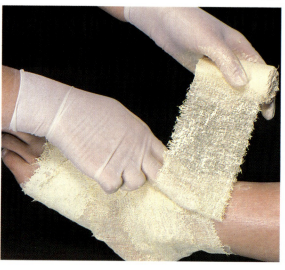

237 Medicated paste bandages are used mainly in patients with atopic eczema, severe venous stasis, and in some patients with neurodermatitis involving the limbs. Many preparations are now commercially available, impregnated with zinc, calamine, tar, or hydrocortisone. The common aim of these bandages is to help the healing of the eczematous area, to provide symptomatic relief from pruritus and inflammation, and to prevent scratching of the lesions by the patient. Such bandages can be left on for several days if necessary. They should be covered with an elasticated tube bandage, which in the case of venous insufficiency can act as a support stocking.

Secondary infection must be thoroughly treated. In severe cases of widespread bacterial infection, systemic antibiotics may be required. If eczema is complicated by herpes infection (eczema herpeticum), topical and systemic acyclovir are often indicated, particularly if the eye is involved and also to prevent herpes meningitis.

Individual types of eczema need investigation and treatment which differ in detail, but which are based upon similar general principles. Differential diagnoses in chronic cases should include fungal infection, psoriasis, and Bowen's disease.

In seborrhoeic eczema, a combination of 2% sulphur and 2% salicylic acid in aqueous cream is useful and often avoids the need for topical corticosteroids. As *Pityrosporum* infection may be playing a part in seborrhoeic dermatitis, a combination of topical hydrocortisone and imidazole creams may be useful in difficult cases.

Index

Actinic reticuloid, 99
Addison's disease, 63–64
Airborne allergic contact dermatitis, 88, 102
Allergic contact dermatitis, see Contact allergic dermatitis
Anaemia, pernicious, 64
Angioedema, 34–35
    drug allergy, 23, 104
    exclusion diets, 112
    food intolerance 109–111
    insect sting allergy, 48
    management, 108
    vibratory, 37
Angry back syndrome, 26, 89
Aquagenic urticaria, 37
Arterial ulcers, 78–79
Arthritis, rheumatoid, 78–79
Asteatotic eczema (eczema crequale), 120
Asthma, 32
Atopic conjunctivitis, 47
Atopic eczema, 8–9, 42–43, 114–118
    contact testing, 26
    food intolerance, 111–112
    hyper-reactivity, 16, 20
    immune mechanisms, 92
    infantile, 42–43
Atopy, 15
Autoantibodies, 30
Autoantibody allergic reactions (Type II hypersensitivity), 21–22, 49–64, 123
Auto-eczematisation (autosensitisation dermatitis), 92
Axillary dermatitis, 86
Azo-dye sensitivity, 110, 111

Bee stings, 48
Benign chronic bullous disease of childhood (linear IgA dermatosis), 49, 53–54
Benzoic acid sensitivity, 110, 111
Biopsy, skin, 28
Blood investigations, 29–32
Bullous dermatoses, 123
Bullous pemphigoid, 51
Butterfly rash, 56

Calcinosis, 59
Caterpillar dermatitis, 88–89, 102
Cayenne pepper spots, 69
Chloramphenicol sensitivity, 83
Cholinergic urticaria, 37, 39
Chronic actinic dermatitis (photosensitive eczema), 99
Chronic idiopathic urticaria, 36
Churg–Strauss syndrome (granulomatous vasculitis), 76, 79
Cicatricial pemphigoid (mucous membrane pemphigoid), 52
Cold urticaria, 37–38
Conjunctivitis, 46–47
Contact allergic dermatitis, 10, 12, 81–90
    airborne, 88, 102
    drug allergy, 90, 104, 106
    granulomatous, 95
    patch tests, 23–26
Contact irritant dermatitis, 91
Contact testing, 26
Contact urticaria, 40
CREST syndrome, 58–59
Cytokines, 19–20

Delayed allergic reactions (Type IV hypersensitivity), 21–22, 81–96, 123–126
Delayed pressure urticaria, 37–38
Dermatitis, 113–126
Dermatitis herpetiformis, 9, 13, 49, 52–53, 123
    food intolerance, 112
    jejunal biopsy, 32, 53
Dermatomyositis, 12, 60–61
Dermatophytid, 92
Dermographism, 11, 16, 23, 37–38
Discoid eczema, 119
Discoid lupus erythematosus, 55, 123
Drugs,
    adverse reactions in the skin, 103–109
    contact allergy, 90, 104, 106
    photosensitizing, 99–100, 101, 107

Eczema, 113–126
    atopic, see Atopic eczema
Eczema herpeticum (Kaposi's varicelliform eruption) 117, 126
En coup de sabre, 58–59
Eosinophilia, 31
Erythema,
    annulare centrifugum, 41–42
    chronicum migrans, 41
    elevatum diutinum, 76
    heliotrope, 60
    multiforme, 11, 41, 74–75, 107
    nail-fold 56, 60–61
    nodosum, 12, 41, 73–74, 108
    reactive, 41–42
Erythematosquamous eruption, 109
Erythematous maculopapular eruption, 105–6
Erythropoietic protoporphyria, 39
Excited skin syndrome, 26
Exclusion diets, 32, 40, 42, 112
Exfoliative dermatitis, 107, 108
Eye, immediate allergic reactions, 46–47

Finn chambers, 23–24
Fish tank granuloma, 94
Fixed drug eruption, 107
Food allergy, 109–112
    angioedema, 34
    contact allergic dermatitis, 88

Garlic dermatitis, 88
Gell and Coombs' classification of hypersensitivity states, 14, 20–22
Giant cell arteritis (temporal arteritis), 77
Gluten sensitivity, 53, 112
Goitre, 62
Granuloma annulare, 13, 93
Granulomas, 93–96
Granulomatous vasculitis (Churg–Strauss syndrome), 76, 79
Graves' disease, 62–63

Hashimoto's disease (autoimmune thyroiditis), 62
Hay fever conjunctivitis, 46–47
Heat urticaria, 37
Heliotrope erythema, 60
Henoch–Schönlein purpura, 65–67
Herpes gestationis, 52, 123
Herpes zoster, 117
House dust mite, 44, 92
Hydroa vacciniforme, 98
Hyperpigmentation,
    Addison's disease, 63–64
    lichen striatus, 122
Hyper-reactivity, 16, 20
Hypersensitivity reactions, 20–22
Hypopigmentation, 116

IgE dependent (hypersensitivity) urticaria, 36
Immediate allergic reactions (Type I hypersensitivity), 21–22, 33–48, 123
Immune complex allergic reactions (Type III hypersensitivity), 21–22, 65–80, 123
Immune system, 17–22
Immunobullous disorders, 49–54
Immunoglobulins, 19, 29
Impetiginisation, 113, 115
Insect sting allergy, 35, 48
Iododerma, 106

Jejunal biopsy, 32, 53
Juvenile plantar dermatosis, 117

Kaposi's varicelliform eruption, 117, 126
Keratinocytes, 19–20
Keratosis pilaris, 116

Langerhans cells, 18–20
Lanolin sensitivity, 85
Leishmaniasis, 93–94
Leprosy, 93
Lethal midline granulomatosis, 80
Leucocytoclastic vasculitis, 65–68, 78
Lichen simplex chronicus, 116, 121
Lichen striatus, 122
Linear IgA dermatosis, 49, 53–54
Livedo vasculitis (segmental hyalinising vasculitis), 68
Lupus erythematosus, 55–57
    cells, 31
    discoid, 55, 123
    management, 123
    systemic, *see* Systemic lupus erythematosus
Lupus pernio, 96
Lymphomatoid granulomatosis, 80

Mastocytosis (urticaria pigmentosa), 34
Mercuric sulphide, 93, 95
Molluscum contagiosum, 118
Morphoea, 58–59
Mucous membrane pemphigoid (cicatricial pemphigoid), 52
Mycobacterial infections, 93
Myxoedema, pretibial, 62–63

Nail varnish contact allergy, 85
Nail-changes, rheumatoid arthritis, 78–79
Nail-fold erythema, 56, 60–61
Nail-fold telangiectasia, 12, 56, 60–61
Nappy dermatitis, 91
Nasal allergy, 44–45
Nasal polyps, 46
Necrotising vasculitis, 67
Neurodermatitis (lichen simplex chronicus), 116, 121
Nickel sensitivity, 83–84, 114
Nodular prurigo, 121
Non-bullous dermatoses, 54–61, 123
Nummular eczema, 119

Oedema, laryngeal, 34–35, 110
Onycholysis, photosensitive, 100

Papular atopic eczema, 116
Paraphenylenediamine sensitivity, 12, 83–84
Paste bandages, 126
Patch tests, 23–26, 89–90
Peak flow measurement, 32

Pemphigoid, 49, 51–52, 123
Pemphigus, 49–50, 123
Pemphigus erythematosus, 49
Pemphigus foliaceus, 49–50
Pemphigus vegetans, 50
Pemphigus vulgaris, 12, 28, 50
Perfumes, 100, 101–102
Pernicious anaemia, 64
Phosphorus sequisulphide allergy, 86
Photoallergy, 92, 97–102
Photopatch testing, 26, 102
Photophobia, 46–47
Photosensitive onycholysis, 100
Photosensitivity, 12, 97–102
    drug allergy, 99–100, 101, 107
    lupus erythematosus, 55–57
Phototoxic contact reactions, 101–102
Physical urticaria, 36–37
Phytophotodermatitis, 100
Pityriasis alba, 116
Pityriasis rosea, 12
Plants, 100, 101–102
Poison ivy, 10, 83
Polyarteritis nodosa, 71–73
Polychondritis, relapsing, 61
Polymorphous light eruption, 98
Polymyalgia rheumatica, 77
Polyps, nasal, 46
Polythene occlusion, 125
Pompholyx, 83, 92, 119
Prurigo, nodular, 121
Pruritus, 16, 51, 108
Psoriasis, 14
Punch biopsy, 28
Purpura, 65–67, 104
PUVA therapy, 26, 125
Pyoderma gangrenosum, 70–71, 123

Radioallergosorbent test (RAST method), 29, 110, 111
Raynaud's phenomenon, 56–59
Reactive erythemas, 41–42
Relapsing polychondritis, 61
Rheumatoid arthritis, 78–79
Rhinitis, 44–46
Rubber sensitivity, 86

Salicylate sensitivity, 23, 46, 110
Sandal dermatitis, 87
Sarcoidosis, 93, 95–96
Scalded skin syndrome, 109
Schamberg's disease, 69
Scleroderma, 58–60
Seborrhoeic eczema, 118, 126
Shingles, 117
Shoe dermatitis, 10, 87
Skin biopsy, 28
Skin immune system, 19–20
Skin prick tests, 27, 110, 111
Soap substitutes, 125
Solar urticaria, 37, 39

Stevens–Johnson syndrome, 11, 74–76, 108
Subacute lupus erythematosus, 56
Sulphasalazine, 11
Sunburn, 98
Sunset yellow (E110) sensitivity, 111
Syphilis, tertiary, 93
Systemic lupus erythematosus, 56–57
    autoantibodies, 30
    lupus erythematosus (LE) cells, 31
    management, 123
    photosensitivity, 100
Systemic sclerosis, 30, 59–60

Tartrazine (E102) sensitivity, 110, 111
Telangiectasia, nail-fold, 12, 56, 60–61
Temperature-dependent urticaria, 37
Temporal arteritis, 77
Tertiary syphilis, 93
Thyroid function tests, 40
Thyroiditis, autoimmune (Hashimoto's disease), 62
Topical corticosteroids,
    contact allergy, 90
    striae, 125
    therapy, 124
Toxic epidermal necrolysis (scalded skin syndrome), 109

Ultraviolet light, 26
Urticaria, 33–41
    contact testing, 26
    dermographism, 11, 16
    drug allergy, 104
    exclusion diets, 112
    food intolerance, 109–111
    management, 123
    provoking factors, 36
    see also, Angioedema
Urticaria pigmentosa (mastocytosis), 34
Urticarial vasculitis, 40, 69–70

Varicose eczema, 120
Vasculitis, 9, 65–76
    drug allergy, 104, 108
    granulomatous (Churg–Strauss syndrome), 76, 79
    leucocytoclastic, 17, 65–68
    livedo (segmental hylanising vasculitis), 68
    necrotising, 67
    systemic, 67
    urticarial, 40, 69–70
Vernal catarrh, 46–47
Vibratory angioedema, 37

Wasp stings, 35, 48
Weals (hives), 33–34
Wegener's granulomatosis, 80
Wet wrap therapy, 126
White dermographism, 16
Wool alcohol sensitivity, 86

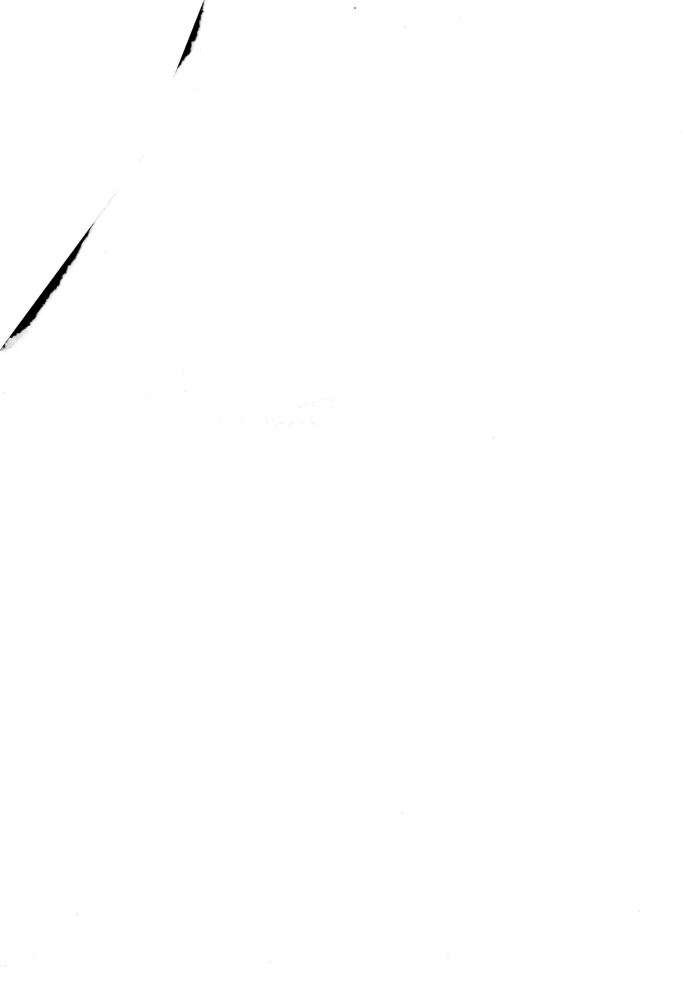